What Professionals Are Saying About
Managing Your Medical Experience

"Dr. Lang has written an accessible and readable book for anyone who suffers anxiety deciding which medical tests or procedures to have, waiting for test results, or talking with medical personnel about health issues. In addition to offering practical strategies for planning ahead of time how to be more personally assertive and take greater control over various medical situations, she provides relaxation and guided self-hypnosis techniques to help people get through situations that are not under their control. An excellent resource for anyone who interacts with the medical system."

> **—Marlene G. Fine, PhD,** Professor of Communications,
> Simmons College, Boston

"The pre-medical visit and procedure suggestions by Dr. Lang are very important to achieve a better patient experience and outcome. Her conversational tone makes the reader feel as if she is sitting beside you as a trusted friend and giving sound, practical and wise advice. Acknowledging the mind body connection, Dr. Lang introduces the reader to Comfort Solutions in a way that draws the reader in to want to know more about the relaxation techniques and self hypnosis that one can use to manage anxiety and discomfort."

> **—Kathleen A. Gross, MSN, BS, RN-BC, CRN,** Editor,
> Journal of Radiology Nursing

"This is an extremely valuable handbook that will be useful for anyone who is planning on undergoing a medical procedure. It is filled with practical and easy to understand information, written by a physician who has firsthand and in-depth knowledge about what patients need to know in order to feel more comfortable with their decisions about medical procedures. The book is filled with clear and easy to use strategies with proven efficacy for making medical procedures easier to deal with and more comfortable. Anyone who is even considering going through a medical procedure should read this book, and take full advantage of the comforting and practical suggestions. A wonderful and incredibly helpful book."

> **—Mark P. Jensen, PhD,** Professor and Vice Chair for Research,
> Department of Physical Medicine and Rehabilitation,
> University of Washington, Seattle

"Elvira Lang is a doctor of extraordinary compassion. She reminds us that the "normal" steps in medical diagnosis and treatment can attack our ability to remain calm and in control. But then she gives us hope. She presents the reader, in a simple and direct fashion, a number of low-tech, but sophisticated, approaches to stress reduction and pain avoidance. Her book is based on sound medical research, but it is written in terms all of us can understand and use. Through it all, you can feel the depth of caring she brings to her practice of medicine. You will finish this book as a stronger and more thoughtful patient, one who can take steps to make your medical experience a better one."

—**Paul F. Levy,** Former CEO and President, Beth Israel Deaconess Medical Center

"Managing Your Medical Experience gets high marks from me both as a physician familiar with the tangle of policies and procedures that are an integral part of healthcare facilities, and as a surgery patient with personal experience of the remarkable relief and improved outcome that these self-hypnosis techniques can provide."

—**Gillian Lieberman, MD,** Director of Radiologic Education, Harvard Medical School Associate Professor, Harvard Medical School Co-director, Radiologic Education, BIDMC

"This book can help individuals understand the stresses of being a patient, and provides practical tips on how to manage the decisions and emotional challenges that come with needing health care. It provides valuable insights into the processes of navigating the health care system positively—for patients, families, and providers. I'm glad I read it!"

—**M. Victoria Marx, MD,** Professor of Clinical Radiology, USC Keck School of Medicine, Fellow Society of Interventional Radiology

"So many patients have told me about the burden, frustration, fears, and often the lack of control they felt as they were seeking information, making decisions, and were waiting for results during the treatment continuum. I wish they could be empowered and use the practical ways so well described in this book. Then they could be dealing optimally with the medical system, and master ways of utilizing relaxation and self-hypnotic techniques in order to remain as comfortable as possible in various medical contexts."

—**Sylvain Néron, PhD,** Assistant Professor, Department of Oncology, McGill University, Coordinator Louise Granofsky Psychosocial Oncology Program, Segal Cancer Centre, Jewish General Hospital, Montreal, Quebec, Canada

"Elvira Lang is a brilliant innovator and compassionate change agent who has committed her career to serving patients. the majority of her career has been dedicated to directly addressing and eradicating patient anxiety. She has leveraged her unique expertise in both procedural medicine and self-hypnosis to change the intersection of these two disciplines, and to deal most successfully with patient anxiety that is related to procedures. In Managing our Medical Experience she takes these carefully crafted and successful approaches, and hands these essential tools directly to patients. Delivering these benefits to patients directly benefits all individuals undergoing a full range of procedures. Dr. Lang's efforts are to be welcomed, celebrated, and applauded."

—**Alexander Norbash, MD, MHCM,** Professor of Radiology, Chairman of Radiology, Boston University School of Medicine

"Finally! A solution to control your fear, anxiety and jitters in the doctor's office and during medical procedures. This book featuring Comfort Talk® will change your life. It has mine."

—**Debbie Phillips, MPA,** Founder, Women on Fire®

"Dr. Lang has written a superb user's manual for mind and body. Built on a solid foundation of careful clinical research, she lucidly shows how to use self-hypnosis as a personal resource to manage pain, stress, and anxiety related to medical problems and procedures. She takes the mystery out of hypnosis and highlights the utility in it. Do try this at home."

—**David Spiegel, MD,** Willson Professor in the School of Medicine, Associate Chair Department of Psychiatry & Behavioral Sciences, Stanford University School of Medicine

"Managing Your Medical Experience is a breakthrough book—empowering patients to help themselves deal with pain and stress while advancing their knowledge and behaviors in ways that ready them for any medical test or treatment journey."

—**Gabriel Tan, PhD, ABPP,** Associate Professor and Director of Clinical Psychology Program, Department of Psychology, National University of Singapore

"Having witnessed Dr. Lang's consistent success applying non-invasive, non-medication relaxation and self-empowering techniques in clinical trials at Ohio State University, I applaud her adaptation of those techniques for patient self-help use. This book is a great resource and useful help for patients."

—**William TC Yuh, MD, FACR,** Professor and Vice Chair, Department of Radiology, University of Washington

MANAGING YOUR MEDICAL EXPERIENCE

THE INFORMATION YOU NEED

PLUS *Self-Hypnosis tips for finding comfort with your tests and treatment*

Elvira V. Lang, MD, PhD, FSIR, FSCEH

Managing Your Medical Experience
is available at: **www.hypnalgesics.com/MYME**

For bulk orders and booksellers
contact directly:

Hypnalgesics, LLC
157 Ivy Street
Brookline, MA 024446

Published 2014.

18 17 16 15 14   1 2 3 4 5

Printed in the United States of America

Design: DECODE, Inc., Seattle

Contents

Introduction

The impetus for *Managing Your Medical Experience*—written for patients wanting to help themselves—grew from reactions to my book *Patient Sedation Without Medication*—co-authored with Dr. E. Laser, PhD. *Patient Sedation Without Medication* was originally designed to train healthcare professionals to guide patients in Comfort Talk®, a non-pharmaceutical process that reduces or eliminates anxiety, pain, and complications during medical tests and procedures. It wasn't long, however, before our trainees were using these techniques on themselves as well as their patients. I began to receive calls (and still do) from friends and friends of friends (including hard core physicians!) who suddenly seemed overwhelmed and frantic about facing an upcoming surgery or dental visit or wanted some concrete advice about making a tough healthcare decision. Additionally, several of our Comfort Talk® trained Medical Center clients asked us if we had any patient-directed materials to help patients become familiar with and prepare themselves for a Comfort Talk® complement to their medical experience. It became clear that patients who were acquainted with the Comfort Talk® techniques before meeting their Comfort Talk® trained personnel in the medical facility could even more quickly participate in helping themselves and had an enhanced and overall very satisfying medical experience.

It was in answer to these reactions to *Patient Sedation Without Medication* and to Comfort Talk® training for medical professionals that I decided to write *Managing Your Medical Experience* for patients. In talking to patients and medical personnel, and calling on the knowledge I have gained over the last 20 years through rigorous clinical trials and testing to find which techniques for relaxation and pain management work well in the medical setting, it became clear that there were two key needs that patients had in

1

managing a medical experience. First: a need for the knowledge to navigate the medical system and wisely make associated decision, and second: a need for non-pharmaceutical tools to help them remain emotionally balanced and regain a resourceful mental state at a moment's notice, as needed. To address these needs, *Managing Your Medical Experience* is presented in two parts.

Part I provides the information necessary to decide on and become ready to schedule and experience a test or procedure. Each Part I chapter addresses a particular challenge associated with coping with medical encounters. In addition to giving background information that helps readers put their issue in perspective by helping them understand why the problem exists, what influences it, and what can and cannot be changed, each chapter offers specific proactive strategies and solutions for managing the chapter topic. Part II and the Appendix of Comfort Solutions provides all of the information needed to find relief and strength through self-hypnosis. Although Part I and Part II are closely integrated and cross-referenced, Part II together with the Appendix of Comfort Solutions also operate as a stand-alone tutorial for understanding and using self-hypnosis.

Being very aware of the time crunch that seems part of most lives, we have designed the Comfort Solutions in this book to give fast, here-and-now support for the chronically time-pressed modern person who may have wanted to prepare ahead of time, but didn't, and is now sitting in the dentist's or pre-op waiting room needing relief. *Managing Your Medical Experience* includes quick, easy to apply solutions for immediate relief.

Liability Disclaimer

The techniques, methods, strategies, information, and opinions presented in *Managing Your Medical Experience* represent the best judgment available to the author based on the data collected during 20 years of clinical work and research involving rigorous prospective randomized studies with >700 patients, and training of medical personnel internationally, all of which clearly shows that the use of the strategies and techniques now known as *Comfort Talk®* and in this book regularly referred to as *Comfort Solutions* make medical procedures more comfortable and safer for patients. While the author is confident that applied as intended these techniques will be effective and safe, use or misuse, is strictly at the risk of user. The author, Hypnalgesics, LLC, Comfort Talk®, and respective officers and representatives disclaim all liability for the up-to-dateness, accuracy, completeness, and quality of the information and for individual application or misapplication of the techniques, methods, strategies, information, and opinions presented in *Managing Your Medical Experience*.

The information, techniques, methods, strategies, and opinions in *Managing Your Medical Experience* is not intended to replace professional medical advice, diagnosis, or treatment and no action or inaction should be based solely on the information presented in *Managing Your Medical Experience*.

The Comfort Solutions can help you manage apprehension and pain during your medical visit or procedure and help you achieve a relaxed state anywhere. Always choose a safe place to enjoy the Comfort Solutions. Do not use while driving, operating machinery, or doing other tasks requiring concentration.

Note: If you are currently in psychological or psychiatric treatment it is important to ensure that there are no contraindications for using the methods, strategies, and techniques presented in *Managing Your Medical Experience*. Discuss your intention to use self-hypnosis with your treating psychotherapist before using the methods, strategies, and techniques presented in *Managing Your Medical Experience*. Stop applying these self-hypnosis techniques if they are not achieving the desired results or you encounter problems. Contact a mental health provider as needed.

How to Use This Book

Chapters 1-14 make up Part I of *Managing Your Medical Experience*. Each of the Part I chapters addresses a particular challenge associated with coping with medical encounters. Together these chapters offer information and insight to help you shape your medical experience to your best advantage and comfort. Several of the chapters introduce one of the Comfort Solutions listed in the Appendix. Comfort Solutions address the emotional component that is an intrinsic part of medical encounters, and provide specific step-by-step instruction for finding physical and emotional comfort through self-hypnosis. Although the Comfort Solutions are related, each can stand alone.

Managing Your Medical Experience is organized to accommodate a variety of approaches. One option is to read through the chapters, pausing to investigate each Comfort Solution as it is introduced. However, Part II of the book—chapters 15, 16, and 17 together with the Comfort Solutions—is a self-contained tutorial providing all the information you need to bring yourself fast comfort through self-hypnosis. Because *Managing Your Medical Experience* is also structured so that you can get right to the information you want/need, another option is to check the Table of Contents to find the topic of immediate interest to you and go right to the chapter and/or Comfort Solution indicated. For full information, follow the cross-references listed in chapters and Comfort Solutions as appropriate.

BEING
PROACTIVE

CHAPTER 1

Scheduling a Test; Waiting for Results

How you approach and endure a medical appointment or medical test is influenced by a number of factors including your expectations, previous experience, relevant background knowledge or misunderstandings, usual approach to stress, general optimism, and how proactive you are. In the following chapters, you will learn how to best deal with the challenges of anticipating and undergoing medical tests and procedures. This chapter addresses the often-underestimated stress of waiting for medical test results. Fortunately, that stress can be avoided or at least considerably diminished if the details of receiving test results are part of your test-arrangements right from the beginning. It's best to consider your receiving-results-needs and preferences even before you call to schedule your appointment.

The Big Picture

As a practicing radiologist, I heard many patients, even those undergoing invasive tests involving surgery, remark that, "Waiting for the results was the worst part of the experience." In my research work on the experience of having large core breast biopsy, where breast tissue is cut out through large-bore needles, the data showed that this perception of the high stress-of-not-knowing is not just imagined.[1]

The body's response to stress is reflected in the way the adrenal glands excrete the steroid hormone cortisol over the day. Cortisol excretion can be measured by analyzing saliva swabs. In one study, cortisol excretion was compared in three groups of women: those told that they had benign, not life-threatening disease; those who had not yet heard their result on the 5th day after their biopsy; and women who had just learned they had cancer.[1] The women who learned they had benign disease displayed normal cortisol profiles. In contrast, women who had not yet heard about their results had highly abnormal patterns of cortisol secretion that were indistinguishable from the secretion patterns of the women who had just learned that they had cancer. Similar biochemical effects of "not knowing" were also reported in men waiting for their prostate biopsy results.[2]

Why is being kept uninformed so stressful? Not knowing implies a lack of predictability—uncertainty, and conditions of uncertainty signal to the brain a need for control.[3] Waiting for the results of a test differs from waiting to take a test. While waiting to have a diagnostic test you can prepare; perhaps think about how to get to the appointment, what to wear, what you will ask, etc. Making definite plans about your approach to the test appointment allows a sense of control within the test context, but once the test is done and you are waiting your control slips. Now, too many unknowns make planning difficult. Knowing, regardless of diagnosis, is a state that is psychologically less taxing than being left to wonder.[4] Tolerance towards uncertainty varies among individuals and situations, and is typically affected by the time one has to wait.

What takes so long? The interval between taking a test and receiving the results varies by test, by facility, and by circumstance. For some tests, such as having an ECG at your doctor's office, results may be immediately available. Imaging tests such as chest X-rays, MRIs, CT scans, and ultrasounds are typically read the same day; screening mammograms may or may not take longer depending on whether a certified reader is on site. Many imaging studies are now also interpreted through *teleradiology*, which is the transmission of images from one location to another—often in other states or even countries—for sharing studies with other physicians and radiologists, who supply reports within varying time frames. Regardless, there is no guarantee even in cases where tests are read the same day that the results will be passed along to the patient that day. Some tests because of their design take additional time. For example, assessing tissue samples from biopsies can happen the same day for needle aspirations, but may take several days if the samples need to be processed with special "fixation" such as soaking in solutions that make it possible to cut tissue into very thin slices or imbibe them with special stains that make the tissue traits easier to analyze. A blood draw might be assessed the same day, but could take weeks if it requires a special analysis that is done only in batches and only once the testing lab receives enough samples to make economical use of necessary test ingredients and comparison samples. Samples might need to be shipped to another facility that specializes in the needed test. Even when test results are finally read, it does not necessarily mean that the results will be released. Results may have to be transcribed, reviewed, signed, and uploaded to an electronic health record file before they will be released. Often these tasks are performed in batches and intermittently rather than throughout the day, which can add one or more wait days. Then the results have to be transmitted to you.

For many years primary care or treating physicians insisted on personally communicating results to their patients under the premise that they know their patients best, and are best qualified to effectively deliver the news and recommend what the next steps should be. So even if you just completed an ultrasound or imaging study and your technologist has a pretty good idea what the finding is, such professionals are typically forbidden to communicate findings. This rule can be very stressful for patients and may cause them to think that the technologist is withholding dire information. It can also be frustrating for technologists who would love to tell a patient that all is okay, but know doing so would risk their being reprimanded or worse. So, not being told what you have in this setting does not mean that there were horrible findings and your probing and trying to squeeze out information from the technologist will likely only make your stress worse.

Do I have a legal right to my test results?

For years the question of whether you had the right to get your medical lab test results directly from the test facility or had to wait until your healthcare provider received them and passed them on to you was mainly influenced by the particular law—or absence thereof—of the state or territory in which you lived; including District of Columbia, Puerto Rico, Guam, North Mariana Islands, Virgin islands, and all fifty states.[5] In mid 2012, only nine of the fifty-five states/territories had specific laws that gave patients the right to have test reports go directly to them. Thirteen of the states/territories had laws restricting release of test reports only to providers; seven had laws allowing test reports to patients only with provider's approval; and the remaining 26 states/territories had no law governing patients direct access to test results.

All laws prohibiting direct access to medical test results were put on notice on September 14, 2011 when the Department of Health and Human Services together with the Centers of Medicare & Medicaid Services, the Centers for Disease Control and Prevention, and the Office for Civil Rights proposed a rule allowing patients to access test results directly from the laboratory. The proposed rule set off debate and the controversy continues, but in early 2014 the change was implemented, and it preempted the laws of the states/territories that had prohibited or restricted patients obtaining their lab results independently of their doctor.

Labs must now give test results directly to patients who ask for them, however, labs have 30 days to comply with a patient's request. The American Medical Association and American Academy of Family Physicians were unsuccessful in their bid to require a disclaimer alerting patients to seek their doctor's interpretation to avoid misunderstanding the report.[6]

The traditional practice of having medical test reports filtered through the ordering physician has an inherent delay, particularly surrounding weekends. If the physician has to retrieve results from a computer terminal, he or she will likely not be on the web all day long but is more likely to do this in the evening or next day morning. Even if a fax or call comes from the lab to the referring physician's office immediately after the test is read, your physician still has to contact you. Unless you have given specific permission, healthcare professionals are not allowed to leave your confidential patient information on an answering machine or to email to you.

Proactive Strategies and Solutions

The following strategies can help you arrange to receive your test results in the manner that best suits your needs, preferences, and circumstances.

Shorten the wait time

Ask questions before you schedule. Find out how long test result generation and communication takes for your test. If it is too long for your liking, and you have other facility options, you may choose another practice providing the same service. There is now a lot of competition in the imaging community and odds are that you can obtain good quality tests with short waiting times even in the same referral network of your insurance. Wherever you go, if you want results quickly, it is always a good idea to avoid scheduling just prior to weekends or holidays, which invariably delay result communication. If a faster turn-around is not feasible or would jeopardize examination quality, at least knowing what to expect will be calming.

Clarify your options for getting the results

Ask what the options are for informing you of the results. You may have to check with the testing facility as well as your referring physician. The test facility may communicate only with the referring physician, or send you a letter and inform your physician. If you have personal voice mail or email, you may want to request that your physician communicates your test results electronically if you are not available to take the call. Some practices now enable patients to retrieve their own results from a secure website with or without prior filtering of the physician.

Decide how you want to learn the results

Once you know your options for receiving test results, consider the following to help you choose which will work best for you:

- Your physician may tell you only the parts of the test he or she feels is helpful and relevant. The full lab report is complete. How much information do you want?
- If the doctor's office cannot reach you, say on a Friday evening, when results come in, your wait time continues.
- People can be upset with an answering machine message about medical tests. Even just a neutral call from a doctor's office such as, "please call the office of Dr. X," could raise alarms in a household or workplace.
- If the test facility allows patients to retrieve their own results from a website without prior filtering of the physician, you need to ask yourself whether you are comfortable reading those results on your own without professional input.
- Computers at the workplace are not private, and employers have the right to monitor your keystrokes, emails, and downloads.

Make sure you fully understand your results

When your results are communicated, be sure you fully understand all terms that are being used. Sometimes terms have a different meaning in everyday use than in medicine and some terms may be purely descriptive and do not represent a specific disease or ominous fate. For example, in medical terms any bump or swelling—even a pimple—is called a *tumor*. Unlike in common everyday usage, *tumor* does **not** mean *cancer* in pathologist speak.

Finally, keep in mind that a long wait for a result means neither that the news is good nor that it is bad. Nevertheless, if you think it is too long since the test and you are still waiting for results, call the referring physician's office and find out the reason for delay. If they have no helpful answer, call the test facility.

Manage your stress

The stress of anticipating a medical test or test results can be challenging. *Part II: Relaxation Techniques & Self-Hypnosis* provides step-by-step directions to help you find sustainable comfort from within. For an immediate quick boost of extra confidence when making the scheduling phone call and negotiating how to receive your results, see Comfort Solution 1, "Relaxation Breathing Technique."

ONE MORE THING...

Ask for a copy of your test results for your records. You might be asked if you want just the "impressions" or "conclusion" or the whole report. Even if you have little interest in plowing through the details of your entire test report, it is wise to ask for the full report. Reading the entire report helps you to understand how a conclusion was arrived at and, yes, sometimes typos happen in the conclusion that contradicts the rest of the report. Even if you really are not up to reading the report now, you'll have it if you need it.

CHAPTER 2

Waiting for a Test or Treatment

The date for your procedure or test is set; now all you have to do is wait. Odds are that although you are busy with your daily tasks, your thoughts keep returning to your upcoming appointment. Some people, after perhaps a fleeting thought on the negative, remain mostly optimistic or neutral. Some others may develop a daily growing sense of worry about the encounter itself or the outcome. The closer the date comes, the more worried they get and may even consider canceling. All in all, once you've established that you need a test or procedure, it is so much better to seek ways to remain calm and focused. This chapter provides strategies to help you manage waiting for scheduled medical appointments.

The Big Picture

There is ample scientific evidence that having a medical test or procedure is stressful for most people. I've had opportunities to personally see some of that research unfold. For example, in three clinical trials that I oversaw, the research team collected information about patients' distress just prior to their tests or procedures in the radiology department.[1, 2, 3] On average, patients reported abnormally high levels of perceived stress and were able to explain in detail the negative impact that the pending exam had on their daily life during the preceding week.[4] They recalled intrusive thoughts, attempts of avoidance, and symptoms of depression. Interestingly, although the patients' tests varied in levels of invasiveness and risk, that factor did not appear to make a difference. What did make a negative and significant difference was their not knowing their diagnosis. For more on the influence of uncertainty on stress, see chapter 1, "Scheduling a Test; Waiting for Results."

People anticipating a medical test or procedure can experience both physical and emotional symptoms that can feed off each other. Emotional symptoms might include anxiety, irritability, anger, and fear.[5] As a result, the heart may beat faster; the blood pressure may be up. These physical symptoms, similar to those of an overload of caffeine, may then reinforce a sense of nervousness and jitter. Depressive thoughts, on the other hand, commonly go along with a slumped posture and slow movements.[6] It's a cause and effect situation with a twist. Research has established that the relation between one's mood and bodily response is a two-way street: sad thoughts can trigger sad posture—droopy shoulders, hung down head, and caved chest.[6] Remarkably, holding oneself in such a sad position signals to the mind that the situation is dire and reinforces feelings of distress. Thus, a self-reinforcing circle of thought-behavior-thought etc. is easily established and maintained. Fortunately, the circle also works in reverse. Lifting the head, straightening the back, pushing the chest out, and/or stopping fidgeting embody confidence, calm, and focus and signal the mind that things are under control and manageable. Keep in mind that loved ones often can pick up on how you feel.[7] Depending on the particular medical circumstance, they may also be feeling stressed about your appointment. Just as a person's depressed thoughts can cause him or her to have sad posture, and vice versa, being around someone who is exhibiting sad posture or expression can cause sad feelings in those looking on. The key is to instill confidence in yourself and others. I talk more about this in chapter 6, "Boosting Your Self-Confidence."

Because the physical and emotional symptoms of stress can cause such discomfort, it is easy to overlook that stress can have an upside. Consider the stress symptom *anxiety*. Common advice is that too **much** anxiety can interfere with critical thinking or even paralyze a person.[8] True enough! However, too **little** anxiety may result in indifference and inaction.[9] So people don't need a lot of anxiety; but they do need some, because in the right dosage, anxiety can propel a person to get up from the couch and get something done.[10, 11] What motivated you to schedule your medical test or procedure? Did being a little anxious about your condition or general health help nudge you to make the initial call?

Fear is another stress symptom with good-side possibilities. As with anxiety, whether that is good or bad seems to depend on the amount of fear the patient feels. Psychologist Irving Lester Janis contends that surgical patients who had too little or too much fear prior to an operation had less rapid recovery than patients who showed moderate anticipatory stress and benefited from the situation-specific "work of worry".[5] These patients tended to collect information on how they would perceive the upcoming events, thus reducing odds of unsettling emotional "surprises" at the actual visit. They also vented their fears, sought communication with their healthcare professionals to correct possibly faulty assumptions, accepted reassurances, and rehearsed the events—all in small manageable dosages. Similar benefits of moderate fear were found for patients awaiting radiation therapy.[12]

The key to getting the most out of stress related to medical encounters appears to have two parts: fix your focus on the process and not on guessing the outcome of the procedure, and work on keeping or bringing your fear down to a moderate level.[13, 14] Not too much. Not too little. Just right.

Proactive Strategies and Solutions

The following strategies can help you better manage the wait period between the minute you schedule your medical appointment and the time you enter the facility for that appointment.

Don't judge yourself

Keep in mind that research, not to mention casual observation, reveals that most people feel stress before a medical test or procedure. Remind yourself that anxious feelings are okay. Feeling embarrassed about it or self-critical is not helpful. As the old saying goes, no situation can't be made worse by feeling guilty about it. There is nothing you have done wrong or are doing wrong for feeling anxious or worried. It is just normal if you do so, and it is okay, too, if you don't. Accept your feelings and take the following actions to frame the situation to your advantage.

Monitor your body signals to yourself and to others

Monitor your posture and expression so that your body position doesn't reinforce feelings of distress. If you notice yourself being hunched over, take a deep breath and straighten up. If your head hangs down, lift it up and feel how just this small movement alone instills some confidence into you, and positively influences those around you. For now just take in one deep breath and think "strength" and straighten up. This small change in posture can often break the cycle.

Rehearse the visit

You can focus on coping strategies and even benefit from the mental stimulation fed by the worries and anxiety to rehearse how your visit will go. You can do this best by focusing on processes over which you have control e.g. how you get there, how you get home, will someone—and if so, who—will accompany you, whom will you tell about it, what do you want to do afterwards, etc. These are topics you can address right now.

Consider, too, the context with which you view the upcoming medical encounter. Not to deny that it is a "must/should/better do," task a self-imposed obligation—but consider taking a look at it from a different perspective. The upcoming visit is also going to provide you a privileged view into modern medicine, and what you will be able to witness first hand might be much more interesting and exciting than any glimpse that any TV show on the topic will reveal. In other words, you are about to have an adventure.

The extent to which you will be able to rehearse your visit is dependent upon your prior exposure and experiences with the medical establishment. You may or may not be familiar with some of the various situations you experience once you have arrived at the facility. I'll cover some of these situations in later chapters to help prepare you for what you might encounter and help you consider which responses may work best with your personal style.

Keep fear at a helpful level

Remember that feeling a little fearful about surgery or medical treatment has been shown to be an advantage and support more rapid recovery. One way to keep fear at a moderate level is to practice relaxation breathing. *Part II: Relaxation Techniques & Self-Hypnosis* provides step-by-step directions to help you find sustainable comfort from within. For immediate calming stress relief, see Comfort Solution 1, "Relaxation Breathing Technique."

CHAPTER 3

Considering a Medical Test before Agreeing to It

When you are a patient, decisions to be made keep coming at you. Initially you must decide whether to agree to a specific test or treatment. Often this first decision unleashes a whole sequence of events. You may have already gotten some information from your doctor and/or other sources, but you are just not sure that you are not missing something. You want answers; but at this point you may not even know what questions to ask and what the pros and cons really are. This chapter provides specific strategies to help you obtain the information you will need to arrive at the best possible decision for you.

The Big Picture

Often there are several options for how medical conditions can be diagnosed or treated. Most commonly, medical personnel explain the technical aspects of the proposed procedure or test and why it is done. Often, somewhat less emphasis is given to explanation of alternative approaches, particularly when those approaches involve the services of specialists other than themselves..

Medical testing, in general, has a positive connotation and is often viewed—in even the most dubious contexts—as "couldn't hurt; good to know." To be sure, when one is sick or has symptoms, having a diagnosis is a first step towards treatment with all the challenges that picking the right one may entail. However, today many medical tests and imaging procedures are recommended and performed for screening while one is healthy or "to rule-out" disease strictly for the legal self-protection of the healthcare provider even when there is little likelihood for the test to answer the clinical question or change management of the case.

While most people might like to know if they have something that can be treated easily and safely to avoid dire consequences if leaving it alone, the reality of testing is not that straightforward. Dr. H. Gilbert Welch and his co-investigators studied the effects of screenings and other presumed preventive measures for specific diseases in healthy people without symptoms.[1] The authors conclude that there is rampant *overdiagnosis,* which they define as occurring "when individuals are diagnosed with conditions that will never cause symptoms or death." Welch et al. go on to say that overdiagnosis is "making people sick in the pursuit of health" and in the end it not only does not save as many lives as promised, but may actually cost lives and life quality. Sometimes what seems an innocuous blood test, such as prostate-specific antigen (PSA), can lead to unforeseen consequences in men who have neither symptoms nor abnormal findings on physical exam. It is therefore important to think the consequences of the test outcome through before having it. For example, once PSA is elevated, the odds are that a prostate biopsy will follow; and if that one is negative, possibly an even more aggressive biopsy follows the first. The more aggressive physicians become with biopsies, the higher their odds of finding cancer cells in a large percentage of men who likely would develop neither cancer symptoms during their lifetime nor die from its spread. Dr. Welch describes the case of one of his physician colleagues who had a PSA sample on a whim, and then went down the biopsy path, which in addition to generating lots of anguish for the colleague resulted in surgical removal of his prostate and lasting impotence. The problem is that in this case or in any individual case, there really is no way to know whether this was a "good" decision that avoided symptomatic prostate cancer, or a "bad" decision that invited undesirable side effects without benefit. Not to overlook the fact that having a "diagnosis" might have adverse effects on one's ability to obtain and pay for health insurance. Thus, there really is no such thing as "just a simple test." It does come down to a personal decision based on a person's willingness to take a risk and his or her need for certainty. How to emotionally approach this difficult quandary will be described in more detail in chapter 4, "Making Right-for-You Decisions." Here we will focus on the knowledge input that needs to go into a decision.

One point that can be missed when deciding whether to test or not, is if the test prescribed is actually the most suitable to provide definitive answers to the health questions being asked. The questions that X-rays, ultrasounds, computed tomography (CT) scans, magnetic resonance imaging (MRI) scans, or other imaging tests can answer are limited by each particular technology. Each imaging test can provide answers only to health questions that fit its technological capability to answer.

One unfortunate practice that promotes inappropriate imaging, which I have observed as radiologist on reading-duty in an emergency room, is that tests are sometimes ordered before a physician has examined the patient; resulting in studies that cannot answer the question based on the laws of physics alone. For example, regular bone X-rays show bones; they do not directly image soft tissues, such as cartilage, a meniscus, or tendons in or around a joint for which another type of study would be necessary. On the other hand, a chest X-ray done in a technique that makes bones less visible may not show a subtle rib fracture. A physical examination before ordering films greatly helps in deciding which kind of imaging study would be the most suitable.

The technologist who performs a test and the physician who will read the images depend largely on the "requisition slip," or order, which should describe exactly what is sought and what the clinical findings are. More often than not these requisitions are filled out as an afterthought and the quality of the exam suffers, resulting in another test being recommended later. Thus, it is important to make sure your health complaints are correctly presented on that requisition; a safeguard is to communicate what your main complaint is to the technologist before the test.

Particularly when it comes to treatment, there are several readily available resources to help patients make personal medical decisions. You may have noticed that brochures or continuous loop videos in an office tend to tout treatments offered by the respective practice and/or have been produced by the manufacturers of devices or drugs promoting a specific treatment available on site. While these information offerings as well as information on the web are helpful resources for the information gathering part of conscious decision making, patients have most to gain from *decision aids*.[2]

Decision aids may be leaflets, interactive videos, video or audiotapes, or person-to-person coaching and are intended to help the patient to personalize the information to their specific situation. Decision aids are NOT supposed to replace a discussion with the practitioner; their purpose is only to help frame that discussion and make sure you do not forget to ask about details that are important to you. Effective decision aids help the patient learn what is and is not currently known about the potential risks, benefits, and outcomes of each of the available options based on the best scientific evidence available.

In 2011, the Cochrane Collaboration, an international non-profit organization that promotes systematic reviews of evidence-based healthcare information, concluded that such decision support resulted in a) greater knowledge, b) lower decisional conflict related to feeling uninformed, c) lower decisional conflict related to feeling unclear about personal values, and d) higher participation in decision making.[3] Incidentally, the Collaboration's review showed that after all this information patients tended to choose elective invasive surgery less than conservative options.

Proactive Strategies and Solutions

The following strategies can help you assess the pros and cons of the healthcare choice you are asked to make.

Ask the consequences of possible test results

It is always helpful to ask what a proposed test is supposed to show or measure and how the results of the test will affect the next step in your care. If there is no change in treatment regardless of whether the result is "positive" or "negative," getting the test is unnecessary, unless it would be psychologically detrimental for you not to know the data the test would supply.

Inquire about your test

When prescribed a test ask how the proposed test works and whether a physical examination could answer the question. Inquire if there are alternative tests and what they would show. Find

The International Patient Decision Aid Standards (IPDAS)

To help you assess the quality of a Decision Aid, the IPADS checklist asks whether the criteria listed below are met. The higher the score (maximally 100) the less biased the report is likely to be. Wikipedia, The Free Encyclopedia on the web has good links to several sites offering Decision Aids and also links to a free paper by Elwyn and others on PLOS One (e4705) that grades a fair number of them.[4]

Check whether the Decision Aid:

- addresses your health condition
- provides information about options
- presents probabilities of outcomes of treatment (positive and negative)
- describes outcomes if condition hadn't been found
- clarifies or expresses values and guides thoughts on what matters most
- indicates whether decision aid was field tested
- indicates how current the aid is
- discloses conflict of interest
- balances the description of options
- bases information of effectiveness on scientific evidence (ideally on randomized clinical trials)

out what the odds are that a test either doesn't find something wrong that is there (a "false negative") or might indicate you have disease that you don't have (a "false positive") and what the consequence of either would be.

Assure correct test execution

Check that the doctor's requisition to the laboratory or imaging facility accurately describes what your complaints and symptoms are so that you get the best possible technique and interpretation. If you have an imaging study, it is also a good idea to let the technologists know what you and your doctor want to find out. Often the techniques are so specialized that he or she can adjust to what is the best technique for you or suggest an alternative test. For example, in MRI imaging, protocols are adjusted for every patient to make sure that the right area is in the best possible view, magnified to the right degree, and examined so that specific tissue characteristics show up best.

Use medical decision aids to assess alternatives

You can obtain much information from your healthcare provider or other sources. Decision aids are of particularly great help for consequential treatments, screening, and preventive medical measures. Many decision aids are available online; just search under the term *decision aid*. To make sure the resulting decision aid report is not biased, you can assess its quality by using a checklist developed by The International Patient Decision Aid Standards (IPDAS) Collaboration. (See Science Perspective)

Deciding whether to agree to a medical test recommendation can be stressful. One way to combat stress is to practice relaxation breathing. Part II: Relaxation Techniques & Self-Hypnosis provides step-by-step directions to help you find sustainable comfort from within. For immediate calming stress relief, see (Appendix) comfort solution 1, "Relaxation Breathing Technique."

Protect your information. When using social media such as Facebook, especially to communicate about health issues, make sure you have checked the privacy settings on the page so that the public, advertisers, friends of friends, and third parties cannot link back to you. In 2012, 4.7 million people did not do this while giving their "like" to Facebook pages about health conditions or treatments, thus freely supplying details that an insurer or employer could use against them.[5]

CHAPTER 4
Making Right-for-You Decisions

You collected all the information relevant to your health decision that is available to you; now it is decision time. If there are several options each with pros and cons, you may be torn between which option to choose. Or, perhaps, one option might intellectually seem the logical choice but just does not "feel" right. If that is the case, you may not even be able to explain your reluctance to the option, but are naggingly uneasy about being pushed in its direction. When you finally make your choice, you want to feel comfortable with your decision whatever the outcome may be. This chapter provides specific strategies to enlist the help of your subconscious decision-making track to help you choose what is in your best interest.

The Big Picture

Research suggests that decision making follows two tracks that work in parallel and support each other. One track—the conscious-mind track—relies on conscious deliberation, operates while the person is actively and fully aware of the process of weighing pros and cons of all consciously available information, and relies on the recall of objective facts and reasoning to make the decision.[1] The other track, which operates while the person is mostly unaware of its work, relies on the subconscious mind.[2] This subconscious-mind track taps into knowledge of how similar situations and possible outcomes felt in the past to make decisions about the most advantageous way to proceed "now."[3]

With correct information and only one or very few variables to weigh, one can usually rely on the conscious-mind track to arrive at a logical decision based on conscious reasoning that favors the best possible choice. However, as soon as decisions becomes more complex, the "gut feeling" of the subconscious wins out in making optimal decisions.[4] This point was well illustrated in a classic gambling experiment at the University of Iowa. Researchers there used a neat trick to demonstrate the involvement of the subconscious-mind track in making advantageous decisions.[5] They had people choose cards from 4 decks—two of which were stacked to lead to losses, and two of which were composed to ensure winning. They used instruments to measure skin conductance of the players' hands to note when their hands would start to sweat, just ever so slightly. This is the same principle that is used in lie detector tests. After having pulled just a few cards from the "losing" decks, the players' fingers started to "sweat" when reaching for the "bad-luck" decks. The sweating was so slight that the players remained unaware of its occurrence. Interestingly, the players also started to avoid the bad-luck decks long before they could express that they had a "hunch" that the deck was unlucky for them or to rationalize why they were avoiding it by consciously keeping track of their wins and losses. The subconscious-mind track clearly beat the conscious-mind track to the best decision.

The subconscious-mind track is not only more efficient for complex decisions but also speedier than the conscious-deliberation track. As shown in the Iowa gambling experiment, one can make optimal decisions and start acting accordingly even without being aware of the reasons behind those actions. This explains why one might have a tough time verbalizing why one wants to choose a certain route. For example, I recall an incident in the surgical suite where while engaged in a tricky surgical procedure I asked for a certain instrument to use. My fellow physician-in-training, who was scrubbed in with me, asked me why I wanted that unusual tool and not the one I usually favored. I couldn't give a reason on the spot. It turned out to be the right choice, but I still couldn't explain why. Only later in the day did I suddenly remember a case from 15 years earlier where a patient's blood vessels were curved in a similar fashion around the area I had to treat and where after multiple frustrating tries I found that only that particular instrument worked. You may have had similar experiences in your daily life where your gut feeling just told you what the next right move should be.

For the immediate "gut feeling" decision method to work well, one has to have had enough prior experiences of similar situations embedded in one's brain to draw upon. William Hudon O' Hanlon, a licensed marriage and family therapist and author, once expressed the idea in a training seminar: "The subconscious is smart about what it is smart about, and dumb about what it is dumb about." In other words, if one has no prior related experience about a situation, one's subconscious mind remains "dumb" on the topic. Accordingly, when I decided to take a chance at repairing the broken flush mechanism of a toilet tank at home, I knew I could not rely on my subconscious, which to that point—in spite of my inside-the-body "plumbing" experiences with blood vessels as an interventional radiologist—was quite dumb about household plumbing. Unlike my subconscious choice of the correct instrument in the operating suite, I knew that use of gut feeling for this task would have been misplaced. Just fudging it or learning by trial and error didn't seem a good idea. That much my subconscious signaled (correctly) but at this stage, it was no help in guiding me in how to best fix the problem. This required conscious decision making input first, as discussed in chapter 3, "Considering a Medical Test before Agreeing to It." I scoured home repair manuals and the web, watched three U-tube videos of how to do it, sorted out what could go wrong and what could be done about it if it did go wrong. The worst risk (flooding the bathroom) I decided was preventable or, should it occur, manageable. Thus remained as risks of proceeding: loss of my time; and possibly screwing up completely, thereby hurting my pride and getting an even greater plumber bill. On the benefit side of going ahead were the excitement of doing something I had never done, enjoying the empowerment of girl-does-it-herself, and not having to coordinate with and pay for a plumber. Now I had sufficient details I could relate to so that my subconscious decision track could weigh in on what would "feel" right based on my personal approach to risk and risk avoidance. (I did go ahead and fix it.)

So how can one access one's subconscious-decision track that knows better? Remember that the subconscious-decision track bases decisions on the way relevant past experiences "felt" as they occurred, and the emotional-body memory was formed. It is this emotional-body memory that re-emerges in a new, but reminiscent situation. All one needs to do is to make this emotional-body reaction observable. That is what "lie detectors" do, and what the skin conductance measuring probes on subjects' fingers in the Iowa gambling experiment discussed above did. Fortunately, such gadgets are not necessary. The built-in, always available, accessible tools to reach the subconscious-mind track are *ideomotor signals.*

Ideomotor signals are involuntary, or automatic, muscle movements of which one is typically unaware.[6] People often nod their head during conversation unconsciously expressing agreement; some may shake their head *no* involuntarily even when they verbalize, "yes." Healthcare professionals can make good use of the automatic muscle movement phenomena to gain insight into patients' inner feelings.[7] Observing a person's involuntary head movements is simple. Almost as simple is formally helping the person to use ideomotor signals to communicate without speaking. One device is to use a pendulum suspended from the person's finger. The person decides which direction (back & forth vs side to side) signals "yes" and which signals "no."[8] The person is asked questions, and the pendulum signals his or her response. It may seem *magic* but it is the same principle as checking on whether a finger sweats more or less. In this case instead of observing the presence of sweating, the motion transmitted by signals from the subconscious-decision track are observed. This method of checking ideomotor signals has been used in medicine and psychology to signal subconscious answers that could subsequently be brought to a patient's awareness and help solve therapeutic puzzles.[9] Ideomotor signals are also used in psychotherapy and during hypnosis when one wants to gain access to the subconscious to identify fears, likes, dislikes, past experiences, and whether it is okay to proceed in a certain way or not.[10]

Ideomotor signals can also be used when one is alert and has to make a decision or wants to explore what one really thinks about a situation by asking one's internal "computer" what the verdict is. After all, nobody knows you better than you do. Why not ask your inner expert? Below, you will learn an easy way to do just that.

Proactive Strategies and Solutions

The following strategies can help you make decisions by enlisting your subconscious-decision making track in your brain through your own ideomotor signals.

Identify your Yes and No fingers

The simplest way to query your subconscious decision track is letting your fingers do the talking. To start just let your hands rest on your lap with your wrist pointing a little downward. Then focus on identifying which is your Yes finger. Begin with a focus on "yes." You may notice one finger wanting to move upward, it may be just a tiny motion or even just a twitch. Follow the same process to determine which one would be your No finger. Just in case, you might also determine an I Don't Know finger and/or an I Don't Want to Answer Yet finger. If the fingers don't identify themselves spontaneously, you can assign roles to them on your own. Lift them individually and sequentially stroking them gently when thinking "yes," "no," or "I don't know."

Test your ideomotor signals

You can do a little test by asking questions with straightforward answers, the correct answers of which are known to you. This exercise can help you develop a feel for how subtle the finger movements may be. When there are pronounced and very quick moves of the fingers, it is usually a sign that you may be exerting some conscious muscle control. By contrast, a discrete muscle twitch or slight movement with a little delay are the best indicators that the answer does come from the subconscious-decision track. To begin the exercise, say to yourself, "my name is (your name here)," and notice the finger indicating "yes." Then pick a name that isn't yours and see what it does. Alternatively, you can test with similar unambiguous questions such as, "the color of my car—or of any object in your field of view with unambiguous color—is x" (which it is) for "yes." Then test for z (which it isn't) for "no."

Use your ideomotor signal to make decisions

You can use your ideomotor signals for occasions when you have good reasons for each of several options, but don't know what to do: "Should I go to the meeting tonight?" or "Should I finish the task I am working on?" You can even use ideomotor signals for mundane questions, such as which shoes to put on or which jacket feels right for the occasion. When you progress to more complex questions affecting your private or professional life the answer indicated by ideomotor signals may sometimes surprise you—your finger signal may indicate, "*yes*," for something you are convinced you would have said "*no*," to or vice versa. You can use the ideomotor signal further by asking, in turn, "is it because I like, hate, am concerned over," or whatever your wording may be for an association with the answer until you have clarity.

When it comes to the very consequential questions of having surgery or making healthcare decisions you will obviously need to have all the information for an "informed" decision as described in chapter 3, "Considering a Medical Test before Agreeing to It," but now you can assess each of the "logical" options to decide whether they are right for you. What's more, if the ideomotor answer is "no" or "I don't know yet," you can ask yourself for the reasons. In this way you may identify which risks and benefits are really important to you and also if you need to obtain additional information. Having the confirmation of your inner wisdom will leave you with the feeling that you are deciding what is right for you. This alone can bring some peace and equanimity.

For further help in managing stress, see *Part II: Relaxation Techniques & Self-Hypnosis* provides step-by-step directions to help you find sustainable comfort from within.

CHAPTER 5
Coping with Tissue Loss

Surgery concerns itself mainly with either repairing tissue— "putting things together"—or removing tissue—"taking things out." Tissue removed can be a minute specimen or an entire limb or organ. Reasons for removal include the presence of cancer or disease, relief of symptoms, and resolution of cosmetic issues. Regardless of amount and reason for the loss of tissue, you will need to be ready to let go and, even possibly, accommodate a resulting sense of grief for the loss. While such a sense of grief may not be surprising when facing removal of an important organ, it can be unexpected when getting "liberated" from otherwise "useless" materials such as infected gallstones, a painful rotten tooth, bleeding uterine fibroids, and even sagging wrinkled skin, which may be excised when getting "embellished." The psychology of tissue loss can be rather tricky and there are, in addition, laws and healthcare facility policies with which patients must cope. This chapter will discuss disposition of removed tissue and address approaches for "letting go."

The Big Picture

The issues that confront patients having surgery with tissue removal fall loosely into five categories: the logistics of tissue disposal, relevant hospital policy, legal ramifications, emotional considerations, and reaction of the physical body.

To begin with, removing any tissue from the body involves some practical logistic considerations. Where does the excised material go? Patient views on removed tissue vary. Some people appear to have little desire to even want to hear details about where it is headed, some patients have religious guidelines about disposal of excised tissue, and some are simply curious. For a variety of reasons patients may ask questions, such as: Can I take it home? What will happen to it if I don't? Can I at least see it? From my practice I recall patients who loved to see and then take home their gallstones that I had removed; usually through a small tube leading through the skin to the gallbladder. I tended to grant their request; after first taking the safeguard of rinsing the stones in cleaning solution. Viewing of the specimen was easy in procedures that were performed while the patient was awake. When anesthesia was involved such arrangements had to be discussed in advance. Nowadays, even without anesthesia, arrangements require advanced agreement because of new regulations. Another popular item for viewing in my practice were the very large blood clots (some of them life threatening) from patients' lungs and blood vessels that I had extracted. These items, however, had to be preserved in formalin and sent for evaluation to the pathologist since the composition of the clots could affect future treatment. Always, if there is concern that what is cut out is cancerous or holds clues to best treatments and outcomes, the tissue will be sent to a pathologist and/or chemical laboratory for examination. These decisions require that a patient sign surgical or other consent forms addressing disposal of tissue with or without explicit statements about transferring his or her rights and ownership of the tissue to the facility. Commonly these paragraphs do not receive particular attention from patients but deserve consideration.

There is much to recommend releasing tissue to the surgical facility. Such tissue is necessary to facilitate important ongoing medical education and research efforts. In a way, such a donation might even provide a strain of immortality. The most famous example of that happening is the HeLa cell line. Its cells date back to 1951 and were originally cervical cancer cells removed from an African American woman: Henrietta Lacks. Although Ms Lacks eventually died of her cancer eight months later, her cells kept dividing and dividing and formed an ever plentiful reservoir of an immortal cell line that is the oldest and most commonly used line in cancer research all over the world to this day.[1] A major issue however was that Ms Lacks was never asked to permit use of her tissue in this way; consent was not legally required at the time. Details about the genetic make-up of these cells, if made public, could reveal health issues of her descendants nowadays. Thus in 2013 her grandchildren reached an unprecedented historic agreement with the National Institute of Health giving the family voice about who can get access to this personal health information and what can be published.[2]

An important aspect of releasing tissue are the intertwined elements of patient privacy, financial exploitation, patients' rights to that gain, and ethical considerations.[3] Biobanks collect human tissue material in combination with information about disease history and lifestyle.[4] The hope is that this research helps investigators better understand disease development and enables "personalized" treatment e.g., identify upfront whether or which therapy can be effective given a patient's genetic make-up. Lawsuits have been fought over whether a person with a "valuable" gene or tissue component ceases to own this genetic information once removed and with it the right to revenues deriving from commercial exploitation of this trait, or at least the right to veto or withdraw consent for continued use.[5] Although ethical issues have prompted discussion for possible change, the laws that regulate tissue ownership currently tend to favor the collecting facility rather than the patient donor.[6]

In general, removed tissue is considered "hazardous" (e.g., potentially infected) and subject to regulations that vary by state and hospital. Legally, it is commonly assumed that once the tissues are excised, the patient no longer owns them and can no longer effect their disposition, particularly once such tissues have entered the research path. Things get even trickier when an assessment of genetic information with regard to future disease is sought. When accompanying a patient recently to a removal of a skin lesion he was handed a consent form to have the tissue used for DNA research looking at the correlation of health and genetic make-up. No further explanation was given and the principal study investigator or representative was not at hand to explain it. In my view the form was unclear in the essential component

36

Do you own your body parts?

In the United States personhood is sacrosanct; one might reasonably assume that such autonomy naturally extends to a person's individual body parts, continuing even when such parts are removed from the body-whole. Remove something from the body, however, and the law takes jurisdiction. In general, body parts including surgically removed tissues, organs, and anatomical parts are *pathological waste* and legally classified as *regulated medical* waste.[10]

The laws governing the disposal of medical waste are anything but simple and notoriously known for their complexity. Contributing to the confusion are the numerous, sometimes overlapping, legislative bodies that regulate medical waste. The U.S. Department of Labor Occupational Safety & Health Administration (OSHA) plays the major role in detailing regulations at the federal level including enforcing their Universal Precautions, which basically demand that all human blood, byproducts, and parts be treated as though it is contaminated.

Since *biohazardous* material is expensive to dispose of, OSHA does list some exceptions.[11] For example menstrual blood in a sanitary pad can be disposed of in a regular trash bin, whereas blood from the same patient, left over from a venipuncture, would be *biohazard.* Additionally, each state has it's own rules, which may or may not closely mirror OSHA's.

To learn the rules in your state, use the State-by-State Regulated Medical Waste Resource Locator at www.hercenter.org/rmw/rmwoverview.cfm. Once you reach your state pages, you might begin by checking the *pathological waste* description under the Definition of Biomedical Waste section. Also definitions vary from state to state. Some are on the sparse side, but some other state pages supply links to that state's statutes and guidelines that give additional detail. For example, on New York's home page, if you scroll down to "Additional Resources", and click on the "Managing Regulated Medical Waste" of continued involvement and I recommended against signing it. Correlating current status of health and DNA make-up might have been okay, but the form as written could also have been interpreted as giving open-ended consent to forevermore allow access to the patient's charts in order to monitor development of any future disease. That would have been quite broad access to privacy and privileged information possibly even to that of descendants from now on. To my mind; much too broad an access to consent to.

Losing body tissue in surgery impacts emotions. Strong feelings arise not only for removal of an organ, which is inherently challenging:[7] even tissue removal during plastic surgery with pleasing results can cause considerable emotional turmoil and grief.[8] When surgery changes the body image, you do need some time for adjustment to the new "you" even when that new you is healthier and more attractive looking. Many medical professionals have this regrettable tendency to identify patients in terms of their disease—a cancer patient, stone case, diabetic, asthmatic, etc. Also for patients, particularly those who suffer for a prolonged time, the disease can become the one reliable constant in their everyday life and may become part of their sense of themselves. Taking then the "label" or "trusted companion" away can cause a crisis of identity. I personally became aware of this most strikingly when I was treating a women for uterine fibroids, benign tumors that had caused her considerable bleeding over time, prevented her from going out sometimes days on end, and led to exhaustion. The treatment, uterine artery embolization, consisted of feeding a small plastic tube from the groin artery into the artery supplying the fibroids and cutting off their blood supply, which lets the fibroids die down and shrivel up. Even though the uterus is preserved during this procedure, and the fibroids were clearly unnecessary, right after procedure the patient experienced a very sudden reaction of grief over losing what had been a constant, reliable presence. Ever since that incident, I have made sure to include some suggestions upfront to prepare patients for dealing with the loss of tissue. Also, patients who have been told by their doctors that they have to "live with" symptoms, may suddenly panic when tissue removal may remove the source of symptoms and allegorically with it "life."[9]

Finally, removing tissue, especially body organs, can have a profound effect on the physical body. Adjusting may take time. Surgical cuts may have changed the routing of nerve impulses and sensations at different body parts may feel different than before. Sometimes it takes awhile before normal sensation returns. The key is to let recovery take its course.

Proactive Strategies and Solutions

Letting tissue go involves practical, legal, emotional, and physical considerations. The following strategies can help you prepare for your surgery to minimize the potential emotional toll.

Decide if you want to see it

If your tissue is removed under anesthesia and you want to see it before it gets processed, make sure you discuss this with your surgeon. He or she may either take a picture, which is commonly done anyhow, or may allow you a glimpse if feasible and doing so does not negatively affect the ability of the pathologist to make a correct diagnosis. If the tissue removed consists of a larger specimen, think through if you would feel okay seeing it and smelling it. Drying blood and flesh is not everyone's thing!

Decide about taking it home

Particularly if you want to take your excised body pieces home, it is best to discuss this upfront during pre-procedure visits—not right before surgery. As the sidebar indicates, there is quite a grey zone on disposition in some state laws. If you express interest, the odds are that your wish will be granted if the tissue is not needed for diagnosis and doesn't represent a clear biohazard. If your surgeon is well enough humored, he or she will likely give you your gallstones or tooth, usually after a quick cleansing rub. If it is anything that may possibly decompose it will be best to put it in a small transparent vial filled with formalin and closed with a non-leaking lid. These items are materials that would need to be there when needed and are not necessarily there if not requested beforehand.

Prepare yourself for letting go

Take a moment to reflect on what will be removed. It can be helpful to prepare yourself for the fact that it will be "gone." Just as with other causes of grief, a good memory, if applicable, can soothe the grief of physical absence. If the removal entails tissue that once was healthy and contributory to your overall body function and wellness, you can acknowledge that. It may be best to set a few minutes apart, take a few deep breaths in and out, and reflect along the line of reasoning presented in the following Self-Reflection Prompt:

Self-Reflection Prompt 5.1

You might remember the times that the tissue or organ, when and while it was healthy, benefitted you and how it contributed to the development and function of your body as well as it did. You may have greatly benefitted from the good work it has done, and that benefit will live on in your memory. It is important to acknowledge the contribution and also to accept that it is okay now to let go. Consider that this part of you, that was there for you, is ready to be let go, too, since in its deeper knowledge it knows that this will further help the whole you to heal and prosper.

Part II: Relaxation Techniques & Self-Hypnosis provides step-by-step directions to help you find sustainable comfort from within. For immediate calming stress relief, see comfort solution 1, "Relaxation Breathing Technique."

CHAPTER 6
Boosting Your Self-Confidence

Whatever the situation, self-doubt can become your enemy. To face the challenges and follow through on the actions you want to take and remain in control you need to initiate and nurture an attitude that allows you to have a positive, realistic perception of yourself and lets your abilities shine. This chapter tells you how to develop that attitude.

The Big Picture

You can probably think of an example of when you wanted to do something or say something and just couldn't bring yourself to do it. Perhaps you wanted to communicate or discuss your situation with loved ones, friends, colleagues, the insurance carrier, or billing office, but you began to doubt that you could articulate your message well or you began to doubt that you would be received in a positive manner. Or you may have just concluded it not being worthwhile to bother. Perhaps you may find it challenging to just ask for help or to stand up for your rights. All of these types of everyday events call on your self-confidence. To move forward, you need to trust yourself to do the right thing, be able to stand your ground, and remain convincing even when the surroundings may not seem supportive.

Confidence is contagious. Research studies show that exposure to another person's emotional expression automatically triggers an equivalent mood in the listener.[1] This phenomenon can be very helpful for families and others supporting a person dealing with medical issues. Because acting with self-confidence can foster a feeling of confidence in others, your being able to muster your confidence can inspire your supporters to feel more confident, which can in turn, re-bolster your self-confidence.

The need for having confidence in oneself is valid in every circumstance. Rosabeth Moss Kanter at Harvard Business School researched extensively how confidence affects winning streaks in sports, business, politics, and personal lives and defined confidence as "the sweet spot between arrogance and despair."[2] In the medical context it is unlikely that overconfidence would lead to overzealous optimistic behavior, but there is a risk of under-confidence, which can lead people to become disengaged, ineffective, and believe that everything is stacked against them. Self-confidence provides the extra boost enabling the extra effort that assures the best possible outcome. Thus, the goal is to provide this extra ingredient that allows a person to focus, act, and collaborate successfully.

Proactive Strategies and Solutions

The following strategies can help you boost your self-confidence and defeat self-doubt.

Don't try; succeed

Whatever you plan to do, don't phrase it in terms of "I'll try ...." *Try* implies that it will not work. Rather say, "I will ...." Or if you are testing options you can say to yourself, "I'll see how (option) works out."

Tune out the negative

If you are surrounded by negative people who tend to put you down, say to yourself "I will only listen to suggestions that are helpful for me and let the rest just pass by." This will allow you to take the emotional venom out of it. In chapter 10, "Neutralizing Negative Suggestions," are more pointers for dealing with negative suggestions that other people throw your way. Key though, will be to feel confident, which will also positively influence the way others will deal with you.

Use self-hypnosis to experience self-confidence at a moments notice

A very effective, easily renewed technique for gaining a state of self-confidence is to use self-hypnosis to first fully immerse yourself in the feeling of confidence with all your senses and then to choose one element of the immersion experience as an anchor—a reminder—that you can easily recall in the future. This anchor can be a color that permeates the scene, a sound that goes along with it, a feeling or movement, or even a smell or taste if they are important to the whole. Recalling the anchor that has been associated with the feeling of being confident brings you right back to that wonderful feeling of total confidence. More importantly, confidence breeds more confidence. *Part II: Relaxation Techniques & Self-Hypnosis* provides step-by-step directions to help you find sustainable comfort from within. Comfort solution 2: "Getting Started with Self-Hypnosis: the Basic Script," (Appendix) provides the basics that you need to use self-hypnosis solutions. Once you are familiar with the basics, you can shape your experience by altering the basic script. For structuring a self-hypnosis experience specifically tailored to strengthen your self-confidence, see comfort solution 4, "Structuring Self-Hypnosis to Strengthen Self-Confidence."

CHAPTER 7
Navigating the Registration Process

Whether you are an experienced old pro or first time visitor to a practice, there may be some procedures that you will wonder about and might possibly misunderstand. This chapter explains some of the peculiarities of rules, regulations, billing needs, and medical practice specifics that you may encounter.

The Big Picture

Registration procedures are largely governed by the privacy and security rules of the Health Insurance Portability and Accountability Act (HIPPAA). HIPPAA was designed to prevent information about your health status from falling into the wrong hands or being shared with persons and entities that you have not specifically authorized to have access. See sidebar for some of the provisions of the HIPPAA Privacy Rule.

It is because of HIPPAA that an inevitable part of registration at any medical facility involves your signing documents giving permission to the facility to access your information and in the course of your treatment share your information among practice members, with other physicians, and, eventually, with your insurance carrier. The authorization of access does NOT include your curious cousin who may working in the practice but is not participating in your care; the same holds true for your sports buddy who is a practice employee and whom you may have been nudging to check out your own medical (or even worse: your parent's) medical record unless specifically authorized in written form by the respective patient. Fines would be pretty stiff for the accessing individuals if caught.

HIPPAA Privacy Rule

If you feel exasperated at the many copies of HIPPAA—the Health Insurance Portability and Accountability Act—information that medical practices and hospitals hand out, take another look. It is HIPPAA privacy and security rules that give you rights over your own health information, regardless of whether they are recorded in paper or electronic form, HIPPAA's Privacy Rule guarantees you the following rights:

- to see or get and retain a copy of your medical record
- to request to have any mistakes corrected
- to get a notice about how your health information is used and shared
- to say how and where you want to be contacted by your healthcare provider
- to file a complaint if you think any of these rights have been violated. One way to do this is through OCR's website (HTTP//www.hhs.gov/ocr)

Specifics of privacy protection vary from practice to practice. You are supposed to be given a copy of the privacy policy of the facility you are visiting, and you will be asked to sign that you received it. Some places may ask you to sign that you were offered it, and waived getting a hard copy. This option may make sense for people having a series of appointments at the same facility over a short period. As always, the key is to be prepared for dealing with a presented privacy policy and have a plan for how you will respond to it (proactive strategies and solutions below offer guidelines).

While the general recommendations in HIPPAA are relatively straightforward the details of privacy protection can sometimes get awkward at reception. HIPPAA protects your *personal identifiers* from unauthorized individuals in association with your medical encounter. These personal identifiers can include name, birthday, age, address, area code, phone number, social security number, etc. Since visitors to a practice are not authorized to access the healthcare information of other patients, you should ideally not be within hearing distance of a person in the registration line who is sharing personal information. Keeping this distance is even more of a challenge when the registration process takes place in the waiting area. Probably the best approach is to make an effort to give fellow patients the privacy you would like. Many practices now call ahead of time to collect your information, which helps speed up the process and hopefully make it more private for all involved.

Even though HIPPAA does not prohibit use of names if use is restricted to calling in patients and no medical information is included some practices call patients in the waiting room only by first name. The assumption is that specific identity is best determined by surname. For example, there are many females named Mary hearing "Mary" doesn't give much information, adding Mary's last name, however, narrows down considerably who specifically is being called. This theory may be debatable if your first name is Genevieve or Elvira and your last name Smith or Lang. The first name practice may potentially also just be the common approach of the many US healthcare professionals who love to be chummy on a first name basis and feel it makes the patient comfortable. For those of European or other international backgrounds this may just cause a shudder, but it is what it is.

When schedule dashboards, which determine the sequence of patients in test and treatment areas, display a patient's name, the entry typically shows either a first name with just the first letter of the last name, or just initials, or only some parts of the patient's hospital ID number. Because any of these formats may give rise to mix-ups, it is always to your benefit to make sure that when you enter each test or treatment area that the accompanying chart is really yours. This holds particularly true when it involves areas where several patients wait together for the next step in their appointment, e.g., blood draws or pre-op visits. In surgical areas this won't be an issue since a "time-out" is required. A *time-out* is a pre-procedure verification process that procedure teams use to review and agree on the patient's identity, site of treatment, and reason for being there. Thus, do not be surprised (or alarmed) when you are already on the OR table and you are asked again what your name is and why you are there. The purpose of a time-out is to help prevent wrong-site, wrong-procedure, and wrong-person surgery errors from happening. It works.

Occasionally, to record your arrival time or sign-out time, or to confirm your having received drugs, materials, and/or explanations, you may be asked to sign your full name on a clipboard list that will remain in plain view of everyone who comes after you until the page is filled. Some practices may blank out your name with an opaque marker the moment your presence is noted—but that doesn't make the practice more compliant since having made it visible to others has already violated your privacy.

Along with the HIPPAA privacy forms, other forms commonly requiring patient's consideration and signatures might include the following:

- Forms authorizing the billing of insurance provider(s), and right along with it an agreement that the patient is ultimately responsible for charges and will pay if the insurance provider denies the claim.
- A photo ID.
- Name and phone number of the person to contact in case of emergency.
- Religious preference, if any.
- Your preference of being listed or not listed in the facility directory. (If you choose not to be listed and someone calls the facility looking for you, the caller will receive no information about you.)
- Healthcare power of attorney in which you name a person to be your healthcare proxy authorized to make all healthcare decisions for you if you are unable to make them for yourself.

It is important to understand that if you are presented paperwork for determining a healthcare proxy, religious services, or to indicate your preference for resuscitation or organ donation is routine and does not mean that you are expected to have untoward events during your hospital stay.

Proactive Strategies and Solutions

To avoid surprises and delays, consider the following suggestions.

Bring all necessary paperwork from home or your ordering physician

This may vary from facility to facility, but the odds are that you will be required to have at least some of the following at hand particularly when you visit the facility the first time: your insurance card(s) including, if applicable, Medicare or Medicaid Insurance card. If you happen to be on Medicare and have supplemental insurance, it is important that you have them recorded in the sequence the billing should occur; otherwise, you may be stuck with greater out-of-pocket cost. Even if the receptionist already recorded this information previously, you may need to produce it again. Also keep in mind that if your insurance changed since your last visit, it is important to have updated information for billing purposes.

Some places may require you to hand carry your referring doctor's requisition slip for imaging procedures. This is rare in the age of electronic order entry but a surgeon just recently told me about the hassle his patients have to go through with one of the imaging centers he has to use. When patients show up without the order from the physician in hand, the registration personnel will have the physician paged, if the physician cannot be reached, the patient will be sent home.

Bring prior films and records if you have them

If your prior treatment was at a different practice that does not share electronic information and images and you have a CD with prior examinations or even hard copy x-rays and are coming for a follow-up exam, bring them with you. Particularly in mammography it is very important to have comparisons to find subtle changes.

Read through the paperwork

Many hospitals, image centers, and practices offer patients the option to fill out paperwork before their appointment, which allows you to take all the time you need to comfortably complete the task without having to juggle a clipboard while you dig for information in a poorly lit, noisy waiting room. Some practices routinely send new patients a packet of all the papers to fill out beforehand and bring to the appointment, others may have a website from which you can download the files yourself, and most practices are willing to gather the papers you will need and have them ready for you to pick up at your convenience. Otherwise, show up early enough for your appointment to be able to read through documents before you sign them. Practices are obliged to hand you their Privacy Notice and have you sign that you received it. Some do this without actually giving it to you. Ask for it and read it through. Should the person behind the counter complain that your reading holds up the line (as has happened!), you could step aside but don't just give in and sign to please. When reading through make sure you indicate areas you don't agree with. Initial, date them, and ask for a copy for your records. Some of these forms cleverly include that you may get mail for fundraisers, advertisements, and possible commercial samples revealing the underlying condition (such as diapers sent to the home address).

Don't sign with full name on publically displayed clipboards

The practice to ask you to sign your full name—sometimes even next to a printed ID or sticker—is rare and inappropriate. If the reason is quality control of wait time and crowd control without medical implications—you might give yourself a nickname to which you will respond when called. When asked to confirm receipt of services or sign-out on an identifiable non-private clipboard, you have to use your real name, but agree to do so only on a sheet that will be kept away from public display.

Inform the practice on possible directives

If you have a medical proxy who can make decisions for you, let the receptionist know whom he or she is and how to reach him or her. Best to also carry a copy of your healthcare proxy assignation with you and have one residing also with your primary care physician; then you can also list your physician among your emergency contacts.

Don't leave home without them

Many medical offices now require co-payments at the time of your visit and possibly upfront at the time of registration before your test or treatment. Some facilities will not accept personal checks; some refuse specific credit cards or all credit cards. Best to check upfront to know how much your liability will be and have ready and at hand an accepted payment options.

ONE MORE THING...

When assigning a healthcare proxy—a person who can make medical decisions for you when you are unable to do so—think beyond the current medical encounter. Spouses or significant others, who often are the natural choice, suffice for most medical events, but they may also be the ones traveling with you if say, an accident occurs and be equally incapacitated. Therefore have an additional, more removed person, listed as a secondary healthcare proxy who could step in should your primary healthcare proxy be unable to perform the service. Keep one extra copy of the form with their names and signatures in your wallet and another one at your primary care physician's office.

CHAPTER 8
Protecting the Accuracy of Your Medical Records

Healthcare providers are required to keep patient records that reflect provider/patient interactions. Such records, traditionally recorded and stored in the paper files of individual doctors, practices, or hospitals are increasingly entered into computers and widely dispersed electronically. The push towards electronic medical records is due to recently established legal requirements to enable better sharing of data among healthcare professionals, reduce redundant testing, and eliminate any errors caused by the "poor handwriting" of physicians. So these days the person questioning you is likely to enter your answers directly into a computer but the odds are that he or she is not the person treating you. The focus of this chapter is to help you understand the kinds of medical records you have, how they are compiled and used, how to check your records for accuracy, and how to correct errors if you find them.

Big Picture

Medical records are the chronology of your health interactions with healthcare providers and include your subjective reasons for seeing the doctor, objective findings on physical exam, your medical history, test results, the diagnosis, prescribed treatment and prescriptions, personal information, and insurance details. The American Recovery and Reinvestment Act requires the conversion to or adoption of such records in the form of Electronic Medical Records (EMRs) by 2014 for seventy percent of the primary care provider population. The Recovery Act authorized the

Centers for Medicare & Medicaid Services to award incentive payments to eligible professionals who demonstrate "meaningful use" of a certified electronic health record (EHR), but they also set 2015 as the year that financial penalties begin for Medicare and Medicaid providers who do not transition to EHRs.

Although the terms electronic health records (EHRs) and electronic medical records (EMRs) are used interchangeably by many people, the Office of the National Coordinator for Health Information Technology makes the following distinction: EMRs are essentially electronic versions of the traditional paper files—they contain a patient's medical and treatment history within the practice creating them. The information in EMRs may not easily travel out of that practice; they may have to be printed out and mailed or hand delivered to specialists, etc. EHRs, in contrast, address the total health of a patient and are designed and equipped to reach beyond the health facility or provider that originally collects and compiles a patient's information; easily allowing the patient's information to move with the patient from provider to provider and facility to facility.[1]

A comprehensive EHR system is required to contain: 1) *electronic clinical information* including physician's notes, nursing assessments, problem lists, and medication lists; 2) *computerized provider order entry* including lab reports, test results, nurses orders, and consultation requests; 3) *results management* including capacity for electronic viewing/storing of lab reports, radiology images, diagnostic test images and results, etc. and 4) *decision support* including clinical guidelines, drug-drug interactions, and drug allergy results. Your doctor may keep more types of records, or may not yet keep this complete series of records. You can review the many advantages of both EMRs and EHRs versus paper records in the Sidebar.

Much of this progressive approach to medical records is good, but there are some challenges. One of the most important is ensuring the accuracy of your medical records. Accuracy is crucial because if there is an error entered by one healthcare professional, that error will be replicated throughout the medical

Advantages of EMR and EHRs Over Paper Records:

EMRs and EHRs have several advantages over paper records as they:

- provide accurate, up-to-date, and complete information about patients at the point of care
- enable quick access to patient records for more coordinated, efficient care and reduction of unnecessary tests and procedures
- facilitate secure sharing of information with patients and other clinicians
- improve patient and provider interaction and communication
- provide a safer, more reliable way for doctors to prescribe medications
- aid legible, complete documentation, and accurate coding and billing
- allow specialists to download your records, hopefully saving you from answering all of the same questions over and over in every doctor's office and healthcare facility you visit.[2]

records system and will be there forever. Another important aspect is that if the person entering your data interprets what you say in ways that do not reflect your true concerns, those misconceptions may also perpetuate themselves in the system. Ultimately, other healthcare professionals may make decisions about your care based on inaccurate information.

As practices change to meet EMR requirements, typically data input is being moved from physicians to medical staff and employees with clerical rather than medical backgrounds. Because the person who enters your initial data is not necessarily a medical specialist, he or she may not catch simple typos that can make your blood pressure or weight, on which medication are measured, appear to rise or fall dramatically with one key stroke. Moreover, non-medical or personnel with limited experience may not correctly understand your complaints. When you finally get to see the doctor, he or she may choose to look at the chart and ask you to confirm what it says or just make a judgment based on what the others have written. This latter approach might raise your risk of being subject to medical error.

Proactive Strategies and Solutions

Being aware of your rights and obligations regarding your medical records can help you protect the their accuracy. The following strategies can get you started.

Tell the doctor or treating healthcare professional your problem firsthand.

Even though you may have already given lots of information to support-staff, it is always medically better if you can describe your complaints in your own words directly to the doctor or person who will treat you. Rather than rolling your eyes and noting that you already told your story, rejoice because having a healthcare professional who wants to know what is troubling you is preferable to the one who just reads off the chart and tells you what you have. If that happens, interrupt and tell your story. It's your appointment, your health, and your right. It will also determine what will be entered as diagnosis and which modifiers will accompany it.

Request copies of your medical records

Simply ask your doctor or other healthcare provider for a copy of your medical records. He or she may request that you fill out a specific request form. As part of your responsibilities, you should know the approximate range of dates for the records you are requesting. Providers may charge you a reasonable fee for copying the documents including cost of paper and the labor of the person making the copy. They may not charge you for searching for your records or retrieving them, and because the Health Insurance Portability and Accountability Act (HIPAA) Privacy Rule gives you the right—with few exceptions—to have access and copies of your medical records, they may not refuse your request.

Check your bill

You also have the right to see your billing records.[3] Just ask. Also most insurers will send you these anyhow. Check them carefully. If you see treatments you did not receive, alert your insurance company immediately. One of the newer scams of identity theft is to steal insurance IDs and bill for treatment and supplies that are not yours. Worse, the conditions they list may label you as having diseases and conditions that are not yours and may adversely affect your future treatment and insurance policy.

Check for errors

When you get a copy of any medical record, check for errors. Especially check the following areas:

- personal information: name, phone number, birthdate, etc.
- weight, height
- symptoms
- test results
- diagnosis
- treatment and supplies provided

If you find errors, request corrections

Patients have the right to have errors in medical records amended. Follow these steps:

1. Write out exactly what the error is and exactly what correction needs to be made to make it right.
2. Contact the provider's office and ask if they have a particular form that you must use to request corrections.

3. Save a copy of everything you are sending them for your own records.

4. Providers and facilities generally have 60 days to make the correction you request. Typically, they will make the correction; however, if for some reason they do not think your request has merit, they may refuse. Write out a formal letter stating your case and submit it. They must, in the least, add your letter to your file.

5. Check your electronic files to be sure the corrections you requested are made.

CHAPTER 9

Tuning Out the Noise

Once you make it through registration, it's likely you will be directed to a waiting room to anticipate the next phase. You might have planned on keeping busy as you wait—perhaps you brought reading matter or work to do, or thought you would browse the magazines provided. On the other hand you may just want to relax, focus, and think through what you want to achieve from the procedure or test. Unfortunately, medical facility waiting rooms, especially hospital waiting rooms, are typically poor environments for quiet reading or reflection. In addition to loud conversations and cellphone use by fellow patients there are pagers beeping, phones ringing, and gurneys and carts rolling nearby. In many places there is endless music and/or television broadcasts at volumes that make them difficult to ignore; and the whole cacophony is likely to be frequently punctuated by announcements over the PA system. When you are finally ushered out of the waiting room into an examination or treatment room, you may be free of the drone of television, but loud conversations among healthcare personal may increase, music playing and PA announcements may persist, and, eventually, you may be subjected to noises from test and treatment instruments and machines during your procedure. Hospitals in general are noisy. This chapter offers tips for tuning the noise out.

The Big Picture

Noise in hospitals has reached alarming levels and ranks among the top complaints of both patients and hospital staff members. The World Health Organization's recommends that sound levels in patient rooms should not exceed 35 decibels.[1] However in reality, these values are routinely and greatly exceeded. In 2005, two acoustics experts Ilene Bush-Vishniac and James E. West published the results of a two-year research project at John Hopkins Hospital and found that not only at their clinic but pretty much

Measuring by Decibels

The unit used to measure the loudness of sound or noise is the decibel, commonly abbreviated as dB. One dB equals 1/10 of a *bel*, which is a unit named after scientist and inventor Alexander Graham Bell. Although decibels are commonly perceived as descriptive of a level of loudness, decibels actually do not measure a single amount, they measure a ratio or relative amount; in other words a decibel compares the loudness of two sounds. Generally, the sound being measured is compared with the lowest audible noise—close to complete silence—which is arbitrarily called 0 dB. A sound 10 times more intense than complete silence is labeled 10 dB. Consequently, a sound 100 times more than complete silence, (10×10) is 20dB, and a 30 dB sound $(10 \times 10 \times 10)$ is 1000 times more intense than complete silence. The easiest way to get a handle on decibel levels is to look at charts that label various sounds. For example, conversational speech is generally classified at 60 dB, normal street noises at 70 dB, and an electric shaver at 80 dB.[G] Sounds around the 80 decibel range are "annoying," those that reach 88 decibels are "very annoying," and the level at which hearing damage, with prolonged exposure, begins is 85 decibels. Coincidently, the noise level of television ranges between 70 to 90 decibels.

Interestingly, how annoying a sound is doesn't always correlate with its measured intensity. Relatively low dB level sounds can cause annoyance when they are in certain environments, such as hospitals where patients may have a lower than usual tolerance for noise.

around the world average daytime hospital sound levels had risen to 72 decibels; nighttime levels to 60.[2] Other studies reported peak noise levels in hospitals >100 decibels[3-5] exceeding those of a jackhammer or heavy truck.[6] While hospital personnel may have gotten used to the ubiquitous cacophony, a newly entering visitor or patient attempting to sleep may experience the noise assault as much more bothersome and annoying. Also, practically constant false alarms on wards can lead to alarm fatigue among hospital staff so that alarms signaling true emergencies may be not be noted.[7]

Annoying or not, the use of televisions has become a waiting room fixture. The standard defense for having television in nearly every waiting and patient room is that it's there to "entertain," the patients. For some patients, that is undoubtedly a realized goal. However, if you prefer to read, mediate, talk softly, or just rest, television is an obstacle, and can raise stress levels.

Some medical facilities are substituting or supplementing commercial television broadcasts in the waiting room with custom made infomercials that promote health-care messages usually tied to products or services provided by the host establishment. These programs are typically on a continuous loop, so if you are there awhile, the message will repeat over and over.

Equal to the pervasiveness of television broadcasts in medical facilities and waiting rooms is the sound of music. In a study in which soft and relaxing music, carefully chosen by music-therapists, was broadcast in corridors, at front desks, and waiting areas, only about 60% of patients, caregivers, and providers actually noticed it; when all were asked whether they would prefer music to the usual sounds about 71% said they would, but 9-12% explicitly disliked it. Ethnicity, age, gender, religion, and educational background played an important role in patient and caregiver preferences; also, caregivers' and providers' beliefs about patient preference for specific types of music were quite off the mark.[8] Typically, however, music is not as carefully selected and rarely adjusted to the patients' taste; and even when it is, the considerable minority who want no music at all are seldom accommodated.

The explanation for why music is played always centers on the claim that it helps patients by entertaining them or by soothing them. But does it? Interestingly, some articles highly recommend music even though the evidence in these papers is not universally recognized as sufficiently supportive of the authors' enthusiastic endorsement. This point is brought out in "Music and its effect on anxiety in short waiting periods: a critical appraisal," by M. Cooke, W. Chaboyer, and M.A. Hiratos.[9] These researchers cite the use of music in clinical practice as a "cost-effective intervention to reduce the anxiety experienced in limited time periods," while noting in the same article that the evidence of its utility is still lacking. In other words, in spite of the widespread use of music, there is no definitive evidence that it works. So why is music played in hospitals including many surgery suites? One simple answer comes to mind: although claimed to be patient centered, the music is primarily for the benefit and entertainment of the healthcare personnel—not the patients. However, there is no firm evidence that listening to music while treating patients improves outcome;[10] to the contrary; there are concerns that it may distract surgical teams from hearing alarms or perceive other warning signs that may not be noticed soon enough.[11]

The perception that noise is not just annoying but can be a harmful to patients is not a new idea. The statement, "Unnecessary noise is the most cruel abuse of care which can be inflicted on either the sick or the well," is attributed to Florence Nightingale and said to have first appeared in her 1859 book, *Notes on Nursing*. Although noise level in hospitals remains a major concern a recent shift in attitude is encouraging change. First there is greater focus on patient-centered care; second there are new policies that link the amount of money a hospital is reimbursed to how satisfied patients are with their care at the facility—and quiet time at night. The result is that some medical facilities are taking effective policy changes to tone down the noise. Some are including formal statements in their Patients Bill of Rights promising to "keep surroundings quiet." Simple actions such as installing padding in chart holders outside of patient rooms, putting up *quiet zone* signs, and holding staff meetings in closed rooms rather than around nursing stations is helping hold down the volume in practices committed to noise reduction.

Proactive Strategies and Solutions

Hopefully, system-wide efforts will continue to cut down on noise; in the mean time, the following strategies can help you reduce the stress of noise and achieve the calm you desire.

Don't assume personnel can hear the alarm

You may find yourself in a recovery room where one of your neighbors has been discharged but some of the monitoring equipment may not have been turned off. When the equipment no longer detects any blood pressure it will beep and beep. Odds are that if you ring the call button in this setting (as has happened to patients) this will not be heard either and your blood will start boiling. You wouldn't be the first patient who then got up to either pull the plug or walk to the nursing unit. While hospitals are making great strides to address the settings of these machines to reduce false alarms—and satisfaction surveys specifically include wait time for response to summons—have a back-up plan of how to get attention when the call button doesn't work. Calling 911 or the nurses' station, getting out of bed, shouting for help or using a whistle may be question of personal preference, circumstances, and urgency.

Ask about quiet policy

If you are sensitive to noise, ask if the facility you will be in has a Quiet Policy or a Patient Bill of Rights that addresses *noise* before your scheduled appointment, if possible. Be aware that policy can vary from facility to facility. If the facility you are in has a quiet policy that is being violated, calmly but firmly remind staff of the policy and ask to have it enforced. If other patients or visitors are being noisy, ask a staff member or member of your care team to speak to them. You may need to visit comfort solution 4, "Structuring Self-Hypnosis to Strengthen Self-Confidence" before doing this.

Be part of the solution, not the problem

As a proactive person, you must also accept the responsibility to not add to the ambient noise. Speak in a low conversational tone and set your cell phone or beeper on vibrate. If you get a call, move to an area where your conversation will not disturb others. And definitely do not answer your cell phone while you talk with the doctor or healthcare professional attending to your needs.

Don't just wait for quiet in the waiting room

Sometimes all you have to do to lower the volume of (or even turn off) a television or music broadcast is to ask. It's a good idea to observe how other people are reacting to the noise. If several people are hanging on every word of a television show or tapping out the rhythm of a song being aired, your chance of getting it turned off is not good and pressing to have it silenced could cause even more stress if other patients object. If this is the case, ask a nurse or other staff if there is a quiet place you can wait. If that fails, ask if there are eye coverings and/or earplugs available for your use. This is an ideal time to bring up your confidence as described in chapter 6, "Boosting Your Self-Confidence," and examining comfort solution 4, "Structuring Self-Hypnosis to Strengthen Self-Confidence."

Engineer your own sound

Another way to deal with bothersome noise, television, and music in medical facilities is to mask it with sounds of your own choosing. An electronic device equipped with silencing headphones and your own audio files can create surround sound tailored to your taste. Earplugs, available in many stores and also sold in some hospital gift shops, may not provide total silence, but can greatly reduce surrounding sounds. Just make sure you let the personnel know that you will not be able to hear them either when they call your name.

Stop the music

In a prep or treatment room, go with your "gut feelings" and make your needs and preferences known. There is no need to feel guilty when you ask to have the music turned off during your treatment if you do not enjoy it. After all, you are here about your health. In surgery rooms the odds are that there will be at least one other staff person glad about your request to have the music turned off.

I am prejudiced in this matter since I never allowed music during procedures to the chagrin of some of my personnel. I personally love music and feel that it would have distracted me from the task at hand, meaning my patients deserved 100% of my attention as a surgeon and they didn't pay the big hospital bills for me and my team to be entertained by the latest rock concert. Also, in surgical teams it is usually the alpha-person who picks the music, and many physicians and staff are afraid to turn the music off (or pick a different tune) for fear of backlash.

When asked as a patient myself during treatments whether I would like music or the radio I used to just say, "no." A follow-up question would sometimes ask whether I would mind, to which I would also reply that I prefer no music. Now I typically say with a broad smile something along these lines: "Oh I prefer to focus myself with some self-hypnosis, this has been shown to improve outcomes." I may add, "Do you need the music?" Some personnel may need the background distraction to function and a surgeon likely will tune the music out when things get critical—but the music still occupies at least one attentive channel that otherwise could be directed to my treatment. So for a massage or tooth cleaning, music would be okay for me; for vascular or laser surgery no—but that is purely personal preference. If the music that is played relaxes you, definitely let it keep playing.

Use all sounds—even bothersome ones—to aid your relaxation

Fortunately you can use self-hypnosis to utilize sounds, even bothersome sounds, to establish calm. Whether you use eyes-open alert hypnosis as described in chapter 16, "Staying Comfortably Alert with Eyes-Open Self-Hypnosis," or eyes-closed methods described in chapter 15, "Using Safe Non-Drug Comfort Solutions" to relax yourself, sound can be a strong ally. Comfort solution 5, "Using All Sounds to Aid Relaxation," provides further guidelines for altering your perception of stressful noise or other people's music and using it to deepen your relaxation.

CHAPTER 10

Neutralizing Negative Suggestions

Negative suggestions abound in the medical setting. With the best of intentions healthcare professionals often alert patients that the injection or procedure about to happen will hurt, sting, or pinch—just a little. Also with the best of intentions friends are often eager to share with you the details of a horrible experience they had when having the procedure you are going to have. Unfortunately, this well meant input can make you feel emotionally much worse about a medical encounter than you ever need to be. This chapter addresses how to counteract negativity, and shape your medical experience to your advantage.

The Big Picture

A *placebo* is a fake treatment. A placebo could be a pill or procedure that appears to patients to be real, but contains no active substance to affect the body. *Placebo effect* is the term used to describe a situation where a patient has a positive health response to a placebo. Testing for placebo effect is common, and research repeatedly shows that in relation to a treatment or drug, positive expectations alone can produce positive outcomes. Therefore most clinical trials include fake control pills or sham treatments to account for this element of expectation. Many people are aware of the positive potential of placebos. What is not as well known is that negative expectations, for example about side effects, also can become self-fulfilling prophecies for patients who receive the fake pill or sham treatment.[1] Moreover, mere words or nonverbal behavior suggestive of an undesirable outcome can cause new or worsening symptoms.[2] Herbert Spiegel, MD describes in the article "Nocebo: The power of suggestibility" an incident where a patient in a cardiology ward was mistakenly administered the last rites (Catholic religious rites once reserved for those in seriously poor health and thought to be near death) that had been requested for the extremely ill patient in the next bed. This mistake of the priest administering the rites to the wrong patient was followed by that patient's death shortly after the priest left. The patient for whom the rites had been ordered and who was expected to die that day, lived another four days.[3] Fortunately, not all nocebo effects are that drastic, but many can be quite bothersome.

The package insert that comes with medicines and the information on specific drugs available on the Internet list possible side effects. Some, such as allergic reactions that interfere with breathing or heart rate are serious and should never be ignored, but just because a side effect is listed does not mean that you will experience it. A list of side effects could be perceived as a list of negative suggestions. Physicians may or may not call your attention to possible side effects; regardless, many patients check out their prescriptions on the Internet. The result of all this information is that some side effects that a patient experiences might be strongly influenced just by the patient knowing the possibilities. This power of suggestion was particularly well shown in a study where patients received a daily high-blood pressure pill (metoprolol), which belongs to a class of drugs that is presumed to possibly cause erectile dysfunction (ED). In the study, the patients were randomized based on the information about the drug they were given at the onset. After 60 days, rates of ED were: 8% in the group that was told neither the name nor the possible side effects of the drug; 13% in the group that was told the name of the drug but not that it could induce ED; and 32% in the group that was told both the name and the possible side effect of ED. Moreover, all patients with ED were then continued on the same metoprolol dose but in a double-blind experiment, where neither the patient nor the researchers knew which patients received the real drug and which received the placebo, patients were given either a reversal agent (tadalafil) or a placebo pill. Patients in both groups had equally effective reversal of ED.[4]

Other areas prone to the negative effects of suggestions are injections and procedures. The use of statements that evoke negative emotional responses in patients is rampant. "I know this hurts. Sorry." "Just a little stick." "This will burn for a moment or two." "This might sting." "Get ready for a pinch." Making such comments is very commonplace and I have found during training sessions with healthcare professionals that it is one of the hardest behaviors to change. Most healthcare professionals make negative statements sincerely and are confident that they are being "honest" and "helpful," by warning the patient of what the professional thinks is sure to happen. However, our research in the procedure suite clearly showed the opposite: Such statements increased pain and anxiety of upcoming stimuli even when the negative warning was modified by "little" or "not much."[5] Other researchers report the same negative effect of such warnings.[6] One of the reasons medical personnel may keep repeating these statements is that their predictions become true. When they predict pain will come with the needle or procedure, the patient is likely to perceive more hurt and express discomfort, which, in turn, convinces the healthcare professional that he or she was just being accurate and may encourage him or her to continue negative predicting—maybe even more so.

Another reason for which some healthcare professionals (or nonmedical friends and acquaintances) may use negative suggestions is the hope that some humor may lighten up the situation and lessen anxiety. Particularly unfunny for the patient was the statement of an anesthesiologist who was recently overheard explaining the anesthetic process to a patient. The anesthesiologist explained he would give the patient a relaxer now and explained what drugs would be administered in the surgery suite, and during the procedure. Finally the anesthesiologist explained how, when the surgical procedure was completed, he would bring the patient "*out,*" He concluded by saying, "...and hopefully, you will eventually wake up," and chuckled. Funny to the doctor; unnerving to the patient.

Proactive Strategies and Solutions

Do not let information negatively affect you

When considering which treatment is the right one for you, it is important to weigh the pros and cons of improvement and any possible risks. Chapters 3, "Considering a Medical Test before Agreeing to It," and chapter 4, "Making Right-for-You Decisions" provide specific strategies for weighing the pros and cons of medical choices. However, once the decision is made, it is important to shift to a positive mindset and move forward with confidence. Should you feel that the package inserts of medications or tales from friends produce symptoms, please refer to chapter 13, "Affecting Blood Circulation and Body Functions," and comfort solution 8, "Adjusting Body Functions and Symptoms to Your Advantage."

Don't try to be funny

Humor in medicine is typically not funny for the person affected with the ailment or about to have the procedure. Thus, if friends, family members, or others have to get ready for a test or surgery, resist sending them a comic card depicting a "hilarious" medical mishap. In this case, so called "humor" may not be helpful.

Immunize against negative statements

Every time you start a conversation about health issues with anyone: medical personnel, your friends, loved ones, or strangers, say to yourself, "I will listen only to suggestions that are helpful for me, and the rest I will just let go by." This is one of the most powerful weapons you can use and you cannot repeat it too often.

Educate your healthcare professional

Particularly when giving an injection, your healthcare professional may say "this will hurt or this will sting, or some other negative warning". My standard reply to this is, "Only if you want it to. Did you know that there is some good research out there that shows that mentioning such words makes it hurt worse?" If the professional should ask what he or she should say, you can reply, "Nothing is just fine." Typically that suffices. For hard core repeaters who start arguing and just keep insisting repeatedly, "... but I know it will hurt" or similar, you can use the following phrase "You are incorrect. I typically experience a delicious sense of tingling." They may look at you strangely but it will stop the negative suggestions cold. It is rare that you have to use the latter—but it has been tested and it works.

CHAPTER 11
Easing Pain

When scheduling a medical test or procedure fear of experiencing pain is often on a person's mind. Some people prefer to be aware and engaged in their treatment; others want general anesthesia and hope to be totally "out of it" during the procedure and remember nothing about it afterwards. This latter choice, however, is becoming less available as more and more procedures and surgeries are being performed while patients are awake. This trend of keeping patients awake when practicable, overall, supports greater safety for patients and empowers them to take a more active part in managing their medical experiences. In this chapter, I address the issue of acute pain during medical procedures and how you can best master it to your advantage.

The Big Picture

In its most basic form pain is a protective mechanism. For example, if you touch a hot plate, your skin receptors send nerve impulses by way of the spinal cord to the brain and motor neurons that signal muscles to contract—instantly withdrawing your hand to avoid further burning. This is a pretty straightforward and useful sequence of cause and effect that is worth preserving. Thus, although patients may wish or ask for total elimination of pain in a medical situation, this can be contrary to their best interest. Sometimes physicians need to identify the location and intensity of a patient's pain, and/or to observe the patient's natural response to a physician-induced reflex in order to make a correct diagnosis and determine effective treatment.

Thus, there are times when pain sensations play an important role, so it is important for patients to understand when pain relief is appropriate and when it is in their best interest to wait for relief. For example, if the patient's appendix is inflamed or if a bone is broken and the patient is on a bumpy ride to the hospital, complete pain relief is desirable and appropriate, but upon arrival

Legislating Pain Management

Appropriate management of pain during medical visits has come front and center of new legislation. Several medical boards now require continued medical education in pain management for doctors, and court cases have established the "right to pain relief." Patients are now specifically asked whether they needed medicine for pain, how often their pain was well controlled, and how often the hospital staff did everything they could to help relieve pain. These surveys become the basis for quality assessments, which influences payment to hospitals by the Centers for Medicare and Medicaid Services (CMS).[13]

In the past, pain management focused mainly on drugs, which can make patients feel drowsy, become constipated, and experience side effects such as impaired breathing. Additionally, drugs can potentially cause dependency. It is no longer possible for physicians to just rely on the good old approaches that were once used to define acceptable standards of care. Recent legal standards imply that "should customary medical practice fail to keep pace with developments and advances in medical science, adherence to custom might constitute a failure to exercise ordinary care," and that "it is entirely possible that what is the usual or customary procedure might itself be negligence."[14] Thus, one may hope that being offered non-drug solutions for pain management as well as medications will soon be a patient's right.

at the hospital, emergency medical personnel want the patient to have just enough pain to help them make a correct diagnosis. This, by the way, is a reason why patients are often not administered painkillers in the emergency room until a diagnosis is made and the need for pending surgery is excluded.

Once left to the discretion of treating physicians, pain relief policies and efforts are now being legislated, monitored, and enforced. See sidebar, "Legislating Pain Management."

Patients are often asked to rate their pain on a scale from 1 to 10. No one event is ranked the same by all patients or even by the same patient at different occasions. Whether a stimulus is perceived as painful depends on its strength, travel path along the nervous system, and the way the brain processes it. The degree to which the stimulus is experienced as hurting is further influenced by the situation in which the stimulus originates, the receiver's general level of awareness, and what the pain means to the individual in that particular context. For example if you experience pressure on your feet while swinging on the dance floor wearing new, tight, but most fashionable shoes or while hiking up and down rugged mountain trails at a picturesque vacation spot, you may consider the sensations all part of a fun activity you mostly enjoy. The same physical sensations in a different context (such the next day when putting shoes on to go to work or during a medical procedure) would likely be considered as unduly painful. As Dr. David Spiegel put it most poignantly: "The strain in the pain is in the brain."

Certain stimuli needles, extreme pressure, burns, etc.—are generally associated with causing pain, but also stimuli typically not seen as pain-causing can produce sensations perceived as painful. Situations where a bland stimulus not strong enough to cause pain under normal conditions causes an ambiguous sensation can be complex. The problem lies in the phenomenon that when feeling something that might or might not be painful, the human mind is hardwired to assume the worst—in this case pain! Also, once one stimulus has been experienced as painful, all subsequent stimuli tend to also be interpreted as painful, regardless of whether they are or are not. Furthermore, each subsequent stimulus tends to be perceived as being more painful than the one before it.[1, 2] In three large clinical trials, we were able to show that pain increases linearly over time during medical procedures and at a rate that is relatively independent of how powerful the stimuli are and regardless of the amount of medication the patient received.[3]

Most people experiencing pain find that when thrust into an engaging situation such as an animated conversation, their pain lessens or disappears and returns only when the distraction ends. Aware of the potential of this phenomenon many healthcare professionals attempt to distract patients in the hope that getting the patient's mind on something else will make the procedure go smoother. One technical solution involves movie goggles and these are starting to make their way into MRI facilities, procedure suites, and operating rooms. Movies can be hypnotic, inducing the person watching to fully immerse him- or herself into the depicted action. Hence, patients' use of movies can be a good idea for some but not all patients during tests and procedures. This approach works only as long as the viewer/patient is willing to give up control over all that is happening around him- or herself, is not interested in peeking now and then to see what is happening, and doesn't mind being interrupted. Furthermore, when an interruption does happen—usually either through external events or the patient's natural rising anxiety—in the middle of the procedure or test, it becomes very difficult at that point to get the patient reimmersed in the movie or calmed otherwise.

A low-tech distraction approach long used by healthcare professionals is to simply engage patients in conversation, which can work; however, there is a catch. Whatever is used to take the patient's mind off the current situation needs to be something that empowers the patient. Pure distraction can even be harmful during procedures when it involves continual efforts to keep the patient's attention on outside events; thereby prohibiting the patient from focusing inward and mobilizing his or her own resources.[4] This practice of distraction becomes particularly pervasive when the healthcare professional is concerned about the patient possibly becoming distressed, having a complication, or being afflicted by an ailment that affects the healthcare professional emotionally. Such circumstances may motivate the healthcare professional to attempt to overcome his or her own emotional distress by overly displaying "mothering" attention, by talking about his or her own personal experiences or vacations, and by asking the patient unnecessary questions. All too often the professional attempting to ease his or her own distress may, without thinking, slip unintended negative suggestions into the conversation. Such distraction is very different from engagement that helps patients help themselves. Such empowering conversations invite the patient to focus on his or her own experience and become fully immersed in that scenario—a lead into the essence of self-hypnosis.

Self-hypnotic relaxation with suggestions for pain control can really shine through all the mechanisms involved in the pain experience by decreasing the subject's awareness of stimuli, decreasing nerve signal conduction along the nervous system, and by reframing the meaning of sensations felt.[5] While there is a place for drugs in care, the evidence concerning efficacy of non-pharmacologic approaches, including self-hypnosis, is growing everyday.[2, 6-12]

Proactive Strategies and Solutions
Use your own distraction

For a quick fix in the dentist chair or similar setting, you might do a little mental math—solve mathematical equations in your head. You can make them as easy or as difficult as you like. For example, work out the answer to 17×21, or starting with 1589 subtract 7 and keep subtracting 7 from successive answers. If math just isn't your thing, you might make up a rhyming poem in your mind or compose a "letter to the editor" about a subject you feel strongly about. Mental tasks such as these can keep you well occupied. Another option is electronic distraction, for which you can bring your own audiotapes, movie goggles, or Google glass. An added appeal of these is that they may discourage the medical staff from attempting to distract you in ways that may not be helpful to you. If you do bring electronic communication equipment, be sure to test and adjust it before the procedure begins so that you can enjoy your program and still hear commands *(hold your breath)* and questions *(what can you feel?)* from medical personnel once the procedure begins. One restriction, if you are scheduled for an MRI, you are not allowed to bring anything magnetic into the scanner room.

Tune out negative suggestions

Since the experience of pain can be precipitated or at the very least made worse by unhelpful comments during your procedure, tell yourself at the beginning of the procedure, "I will listen only to suggestions that are helpful for me." For more on protecting yourself from negative suggestions see chapter 10, "Neutralizing Negative Suggestions."

Use the Comfort Solutions

Comfort solution 6, "Finding Comfort," includes two clinically tested self-hypnosis scripts for your personal use to address potentially painful stimuli during medical procedures. Option 1 script includes suggestions to help you focus on sensations in a part of the body other than the one experiencing pain—a technique that you may be able to use by itself. This technique is quite straightforward. For example, rubbing your thumb and forefinger together and focusing on all the fine sensations that come along with this simple movement may be all you need to do to feel better. Or you may focus on curling your toes individually one after the other. Option 2 script helps you visualize a stone gently floating in water to reach successively greater levels of relief and comfort. You can also choose to just "dial" the pain down. Comfort solution, 8, "Adjusting Body Functions and Symptoms to Your Advantage" includes directions for "dialing" down your pain. Sometimes just reducing the hurt from gradually from high to manageable may be all that's needed.

CHAPTER 12
Soothing Anxiety

Anxiety is a person's response to a perceived threat. Pretty much everyone feels anxiety now and then, but what triggers anxiety varies from person-to-person, and circumstance-to-circumstance. Also, the degree of intensity felt by any person can vary greatly by incident. Although anxiety is typically classified as negative, in times of uncertainty anxiety can be beneficial provided it is in the right amount: not so much that it overtakes one's thinking nor so little that it allows one to become inappropriately complacent. For more on the positive aspect of anxiety, see chapter 2, "Waiting for a Test or Treatment." In this chapter I focus on conquering one's emotions when, in the context of medial tests and treatments, anxiety and worries flare up and need to be controlled.

The Big Picture

Medical literature typically measures anxiety in terms of baseline trait anxiety (which reflects a person's general anxiety-related personality characteristic) and state anxiety (which reflects a person's level of anxiety surrounding a specific event) to arrive at a combination of the person's general disposition and the effect of the superimposed event. For many people, medical encounters may be perceived as a threat and, therefore, can trigger elevated state anxiety, which is the focus of this chapter.[1] In this book, reference to anxiety, unless stated otherwise, refers to state anxiety, and while our focus is on managing state anxiety related to medical encounters, the strategies presented may transfer to non-medical settings of more or less stress. If you have abnormally high trait anxiety or an anxiety disorder you should consult your healthcare provider.

Anxiety can express itself by feelings of apprehension, tension, nervousness, or worries. Research studies have shown that during medical procedures under standard care conditions, anxiety tends to increase linearly over time regardless of the amount of drugs given.[2-4] In contrast, when patients are read a self-hypnotic relaxation script at the onset of their medical procedures, their anxiety quickly decreases and remains well controlled. Research data demonstrates that patients who enter the medical procedure room with high anxiety levels tend to have more pain and also receive nearly double the amount of drugs than less anxious patients receive. What's more, the procedures of highly anxious patients typically take significantly longer.[5] Interestingly, among patients who had a self-hypnosis script read to them at the beginning of a medical procedure, those patients who initially had the highest levels of anxiety experienced the greatest decrease in their anxiety during the procedure. Patients with low anxiety levels at the onset coped relatively well whether left to their own devices or read the self-hypnosis script. The study conclusion: it pays to have one's anxiety well managed before arriving in the procedure room.

In the study described above, patients had control over the amount of medication they received. When patients felt a need for medication relief they signaled their request by ringing a bell or by asking caregivers for medication. Such autonomy is not always given to patients, and overall, the amount of drugs given during medical procedures varies strongly, depending more on the customs of the institution rather than on the needs of the patient.[6] When surveying what drives personnel to administer sedation drugs to patients, we found that staff concerns that a patient *might be* or *might become* anxious was top on of the list; suggesting that drugs are often given when a patient does not yet need them.[6] Second on the list was evident anxiety.

Unfortunately, giving a patient drugs when there is no clinical need or giving them for something that could be managed without drugs can evolve into the situation where the patient later does need drugs to manage pain and anxiety, but can no longer receive them. The reason for the restriction is that relaxation-drugs and pain-drugs are typically given in combination, since they enhance each other's effect. Both types of drug also depress breathing and blood pressure, and these side effects linger longer than the drug's ability to relief pain. When pain or anxiety develops after the prophylactic drug administration has already depressed breathing and/or blood pressure, it becomes unsafe to administer additional drugs unless a breathing tube is inserted.

The best approach to anxiety management depends on the feelings that go along with the anxiety. Sometimes anxiety is an ill-defined feeling of threat or panic; or the imagination may go wild and come up with unrealistic worst-case scenarios—*I will be an invalid, unable to do anything; I will starve if nobody comes to visit me or they will put me in a nursing home and I will never get back home.* Things become more manageable when these ill-defined fears are translated into specific concerns or issues at hand such as—*the cast on my leg will keep me from going up and down the stairs, I won't be able to drive my car to the grocery store, and my family is out of town.* This more specific phrasing can help you boil down your key concerns, which in this example are *I need a way to get food and I need someone to look after me.* Framing the problem in terms of specific needs facilitates generation of solutions for the bothering thoughts. For example, if a leg cast is anticipated, you might decide to educate yourself about how to use crutches and have them fit properly or you might secure a walker or wheelchair for home use. If food provision is an issue you might think about arranging delivery from a grocery store or from a community meal service. If being left alone is a concern, you might give the house key to a trusted person and ask him or her to check on you, or you might purchase a medical alert system, or, at the very least, arrange to have a functioning telephone or cell phone (plus charger) at your bedside. Making realistic plans about concrete issues usually helps quell overall anxiety.

Proactive Strategies and Solutions

When anxiety shows itself mainly in the form of distressing thoughts, you can best manage it by reframing the meaning of the problem and/or moving the bothersome thoughts outside your head for more objective viewing and easier design of appropriate solutions. You will find some of these techniques below and also in comfort solution 7, "Taming Anxiety and Worries." If your anxiety manifests itself mainly in the form of physical symptoms such as a racing heart or elevated blood pressure, refer to comfort solution 8, "Adjusting Body Functions and Symptoms to Your Advantage."

Rephrase ill-defined fears in terms of worries or concerns

Spelling out what the problem is in terms of concrete concerns acknowledges the feeling but takes the emotional venom out of it, allowing you to work out solutions. Defining problems shifts the approach from a passive vague feeling that can be overwhelming to active problem solving.

Be curious and excited

Max Shapiro, PhD, an experienced hypnotherapist and director of education of the New England Society of Hypnosis, phrased it very well, "Curiosity is THE antidote to anxiety." Thus, I often make an effort to encourage surgery patients waiting for their procedures to take an interest in the environment and attempt to excite them about being privileged to such an insider view of a hospital's workings—much better than any of the scenes depicted in ER or hospital movies and soap operas. Suggesting excitement and curiosity is a departure from the traditional advice of, "calm down." Harvard Business School has also adopted this new approach for managing performance anxiety.[7] Allison Wood Brooks of Harvard Business School conducted experiments and concluded, "Keep calm and carry on" is not the best way to cope; reappraising the feeling as exciting and simply affirming that to oneself by saying, "I am excited" reduces the dread and improves subsequent performance.

Make a deal with the anesthesiologist or sedation nurse

Consider how you want to experience your medical procedure upfront and how you will communicate to the professional who is responsible for your comfort. Explain that you want to be involved in the amount of drugs you receive and expect to be asked before they are administered and that you wish to remain alert (if that is what you want). You can also explain that you are good at self-hypnosis and that you would like to enter this procedure in a partnership. Some patients have reported to me that they had their anesthesiologist agree to such a deal and then still knocked them out cold with the first injection. This is fortunately rare and saying that you will check the chart afterwards to see if the anesthesiologist kept his or her word may be an extra incentive for that not to occur. Do check the chart and if it does happen, report the incident to the hospital and medical board.

Be more present in the moment

There is a human tendency to catastrophize, in other words to view and describe a situation as much worse than it actually is. When engaged in catastrophizing and dwelling on the imagined dire future, one tends to forget the actual present. To paraphrase Jon Kabot Zinn, internationally known scientist and meditation teacher, *this moment is the only life you have, and it is now.*[8] Managing a medical experience may extend beyond one's own experience to that of loved ones. I could sit across from my husband and bemoan his progressively and rapidly failing memory and mourn all that is lost compared to the character of past conversations. On the other hand, when I reflect on the requirements of meaningful human interactions, I ask myself how often does one talk about rocket science, how much does one need to remember history or construct the predictable future in the moment; and even, is it necessary to understand all the subtleties of what is said to find satisfaction in the conversation. Just being there in the moment can have magic—provided one lives it with awareness.

ONE MORE THING...

If you are one of the people who tend to imagine the very worst, there is good news for you: This imaginative ability makes you also exquisitely suited to use self-hypnotic techniques to overcome such states of heightened anxiety.[9] So—there is at least one thing less to worry about.

CHAPTER 13
Affecting Blood Circulation and Body Functions

If you are a patient in the hospital or visiting a facility for an outpatient procedure, the medical staff will keep an eye on your body's basic functions by monitoring your *vital signs*. The four main vital signs are body temperature, blood pressure, heart rate (pulse), and breathing rate (respiration). Regardless of your diagnosis and treatment plan, you will feel most comfortable and your body will heal better and faster if all of your general physiology is in sync and working optimally. Physiology in this context includes any mechanism that affects how fast your heart beats, how often and deep you breathe, how rapidly your intestines push the food along, how tight your stomach feels, how much blood supply gets into your fingertips, and/or how well you fight infections. While many of these functions typically work automatically, it's important to know which factors might affect them and how you can deliberately influence them.

The Big Picture

A lot of fine-tuned regulation of the body is going on all the time with multiple mechanisms holding each other in check so that ideally there are no occurrences of having too much or too little of any mechanism. Normally, in wellness, these systems work just right—the immune system is neither too weak for fighting infections nor so overactive that it attacks the body; the respiratory system regulates breathing so inbreaths come just often and deep enough to get all the oxygen the body needs for any given situation; and outbreaths release carbon dioxide without overdoing it and blowing so much carbon dioxide out of the lungs that the resultant low-levels in the blood make a person lightheaded; the stomach "knows" just how much hydrochloric acid to add to the food for digestion without causing gastritis; and the gut does its job without producing diarrhea nor constipation. All of these precise body function adjustments happen most of the time without us thinking about them consciously. What's more, even the body functions over which there is some conscious control—such as muscle movements—involve a lot of subconscious action. For example, to stand straight even for a few moments requires a lot of coordination within the muscles of the legs, calves, back, and arms. Muscles on the front, back, and sides have to coordinate with each other, twitching in rhythm to keep the body upright. Yes, you can consciously decide to sway back and forth but your body just knows how to do this with minute adjustments without your having to consciously adapt.

The body also precisely adjusts the muscle tension in individual muscles depending on whether the body is on a flat, inclining, or declining surface, which means that there is not one ideal muscle tension for each muscle but, rather, an appropriate tension for a given situation. In the same way there is not one ideal heart rate or blood pressure for all situations. When you run or walk up several flights of stairs your heart has to beat faster and you have to breathe faster to accommodate the extra work. When it is hot enough that you are at risk of overheating, the smallest blood vessels in your hands need to open up more to let the extra heat dissipate; in contrast, when it is cold the same blood vessels clamp down to keep as much of the warm blood in the core of the body where it counts most to keep you safe. The subconscious mind is geared to keep the body balanced in order to keep it safe and functioning and as long as all works well, people typically do not become aware of these automatic, so called *autonomic functions*. When stressed, however, the additional input from the brain can shake that fragile balance.

There are situations where changes in physiology happen out of proportion to a given level of activity and physical environment.

One example is the so called "white coat syndrome," named for the phenomenon where sudden focus on discomfort and/or anxiety cause a person's blood pressure to rise merely by entering the doctor's office. Other examples are performance anxiety; getting all red cheeks for feeling ashamed; or the proverbial situation in which one wets one's pants. Thus, in the interaction between feelings and physiologic function, the feeling becomes the driver to

Biofeedback

Biofeedback is a technique for showing the interaction between mind and body function and can be used to support relaxation. Some people who apply their thoughts to calm themselves enjoy getting objective demonstration of how effective their efforts are, and biofeedback provides precise feedback. For many others the main value lies in becoming actually aware of how stressed they are and learning to listen to their body again by getting external prompts from a feedback device. The feedback comes from sensors that are attached to or contact different parts of the body during a session. The sensors show the user information about physiologic activities such as brain waves, heart function, muscle activity, and skin temperature. The feedback comes to the subject in visual or auditory cues, such as blinking lights, beeping sounds, or images in different colors.

The basic mechanism is that by changing your thoughts and/or emotions you affect physical changes in your body and the feedback device shows you in which direction they are going. The ultimate goal is to develop enough body awareness and mastery in reliably influencing body function that the external feedback device becomes superfluous. For that to occur it may take many sessions. Be aware that biofeedback training programs, biofeedback practitioners, and biofeedback devices vary in format, effectiveness, and reputability. Check with your doctor before investing.

produce an unhelpful outcome. There are techniques, however, for harnessing this power of the mind over *autonomic* functions to adjusting functions to your advantage. One example of this is *biofeedback* (see sidebar).

Simply being engaged in a state of relaxation, meditation, or self-hypnosis has been shown to stabilize vital signs. The good news is that self-hypnotic relaxation can work anywhere—even at the height of medical procedures—to keep blood pressure and heart rate in a more normal range, thus avoiding large swings that might result in fainting or other complications.[1, 2, 3] One of the hypotheses that underlie the working of mind-body interventions in syncing body function is their effect on the fine-tuning ability of the organism that keep the vascular system stable overall.[4, 5] Such improved "heart-rate variability" profiles have been associated with better medical outcomes in general.[6, 7] You can learn how to enter such a state in chapter 15, "Using Safe Non-Drug Comfort Solutions."

Proactive Strategies and Solutions

Your vital signs and other physiology assessments obtained by healthcare professionals are used to classify your condition and may become the basis for medical decisions about your care. Knowing what affects your blood circulation and other body functions can help you gage the relevance of measurements that are obtained in the office.

Make sure office measurements reflect your every day vital signs

When medications are adjusted to the measurements obtained at the time of the doctor's visit and you feel that this is not how your vital sign behave at home, express your concerns. In particular for selection of blood pressure medication checks at home in different body positions will be important to assure that you are neither over- nor under-medicated.

Use your mind to affect physiology

Being aware of how you can consciously affect your physiology, might help you attain the most healthful levels for you. This can come in handy particularly when stress provokes or worsens unpleasant symptoms, for example if you are in the dentist's waiting room and hearing the drill makes your heart beat faster and your stomach turn in a knot. For such settings see comfort solution 8, "Adjusting Body Functions and Symptoms to Your Advantage," which provides guidelines and safe actions to help you affect your blood circulation and body functions. Managing medical symptoms with mind-body approaches otherwise should never be done without physician advice. In emergencies, however, there are self-hypnosis techniques that you can use to improve your status until the ambulance arrives or needed drugs are available If it turns out that your symptoms have sufficiently resolved by the time the ambulance arrives, all the better—but you will still need medical attention to make sure that you have nor let a beginning stroke or heart attack left unnoticed. The important point to remember is that for emergencies first call 911 and/or use what your physician prescribed; after that, consider the techniques presented in comfort solution 8, "Adjusting Body Functions and Symptoms to Your Advantage."

CHAPTER 14

Aiding Healing and Recovery

You have a lot to be proud of because just being at this stage in your medical experience means you managed your way through the waiting and decision-making of the diagnostic stage, and went on to accept the treatment. Now, as you enter the healing and recovery stage, the main challenge for you is to balance rest and activity. You need to give your body enough rest to recover, yet be active enough to prevent complications. You also need to balance your expectations. You may need to work hard, patiently and positively on restoring body function while also having to avoid overdoing it and/or becoming discouraged. This chapter aims to prepare you for what you might experience and how to proceed as smoothly as possible to a healthier self.

The Big Picture

Recovery pretty much starts at the time of surgery and is greatly aided by all the preparations you may have already undertaken. The benefits of self-hypnotic techniques before and during treatment carry over into the recovery period and prepare you for restoration of normal body functions. For specific suggestions you can refer to comfort solution 9, "Suggestions for Healing and Recovery."

Needs and circumstances after treatment vary according to the procedure performed and a person's general physical and mental state. Some common situations are discussed below.

Immediately after major surgery, tissue manipulation, or dental interventions the way you feel may make you wonder whether going through all this was such a good idea. Be assured though that the healing process follows an exponential curve, in other words, there is very dramatic improvement from one day to the next, sometimes even from one hour to the next.

It is important to keep in mind that you don't have to prove anything to yourself or anybody else: Perhaps you have become quite adept at applying some of the hypnotic techniques presented in this book and have used them successfully in preparing for your treatment and/or during your procedure. If so, you can call on them again to help you through the healing stage. However, there may be times when you may need to take a painkiller to get you over the initial recovery stages after surgery or dentistry. As pointed out in comfort solution 6, "Finding Comfort," above all, do not feel guilty if you are not completely pain free. The goal is to take the hurt out of the pain. If you do need some medication it is perfectly okay to take it. The research of our clinical trials showed that taking analgesics (drugs that relieve pain) doesn't interfere with a person's ability to gain benefit from self-hypnosis. The literature on acute pain management also acknowledges that it is better to take the medication early on rather than waiting until your pain tolerance has maxed out. This latter practice (sometimes referred to as "chasing the pain,") overall requires much more of the drug to achieve relief. In contrast, you may also find that sometimes just a single dose early on calms things down sufficiently so that further medication may not be required.

The fundamental care goal in the early post-operative period is prevention of complications; blood clots that form in the legs and travel to the lungs are especially feared. Because immobility is the common cause of such blood clots, your medical team may chase you out of bed much earlier than you might expect; often earlier than you might have done on your own. When the risk of blood clots is high, patients may also be given blood-thinning drugs. After surgeries or with prolonged bed rest, you may be given an "incentive spirometer" a small contraption with a mouthpiece into which you breathe with the goal of moving a little ball or other marker to a predetermined spot. This device is a lifesaver because it helps to keep the lungs well aerated so that they don't become a breeding ground for infections. During this early stage, as well as the following stage of physical rehabilitation, self-hypnotic comfort management can be particularly helpful. As pointed out in chapter 16, "Staying Comfortably Alert with Eyes-Open Self-Hypnosis," self-hypnosis doesn't require closed eyes and inactivity; it works equally well with eyes open and during activity. Clinical trials with objective outcome measurements have shown that continued engagement in self-hypnosis speeds the healing of wounds and bone.[1, 2]

It is important for patients and caregivers to acknowledge that treatment can challenge body reserves and that some tender loving care is in order to aid recovery. Patients who have radiation, chemotherapy, some image-guided procedures, or other treatment that may not to show any major outside marks of interventions are particularly likely to rebuff the need for recuperation—a reaction not in their own best interest. To be clear, my advice here is not to stay in bed all day, but rather to pursue a gentle healthy daily routine. Champions of recovery could be eating a healthful diet, exercising (walking; although you might be only able to move your arms, do toe raises, or move your legs around at first) as much a possible, stopping smoking, taking short power naps, or short relaxation breaks—even if just for a few minutes. Patience and moderation are other champions of recovery—as is overcoming the urge to immediately take care of all the tasks that accumulated prior to treatment. This is not the time to redecorate the house or fill every moment with work-related tasks. Key also is not to be discouraged when fatigue sets in earlier than expected. The recovery stage is a time to respect your body and work with it; not fight against it.

Nagging impediments to recovery may emerge if there is some ambiguity about your getting well again. Furthermore, your doctor may have unwittingly implanted some negative suggestions that make you believe that you should feel pain or have other unfavorable effects. For more information on the risks of negative suggestions, see chapter 10, "Neutralizing Negative Suggestions."

Another source of impediments to recovery is unrealistic expectations. You may have been given such through the advertisement industry possibly by way of the educational/ promotional pamphlets distributed by your healthcare providers. These messages tend to overstate, and may have promised that you will be happy forever after having the nose job, or will be able to immediately run a marathon, which you weren't able to do even when your knees were still perfectly healthy. Finally, if your treatment involved loss of tissue, you may still need to resolve your emotional reaction to the tissue loss. For help with this challenge, see chapter 5, "Coping with Tissue Loss."

Proactive Strategies and Solutions

The Comfort Solutions in Part II can help you utilize self-hypnotic techniques for general relaxation, and to address specific needs including relieving pain and anxiety.

Use positive suggestions before, during, and after your treatment

Even before you enter or complete your surgery, you can promote the quick return of your body functions to a healthy normal state, restore your appetite, move your bowels, and start your tissue healing by using comfort solution 9, "Suggestions for Healing and Recovery." Throughout recovery you can use chapter 17, "Integrating Helpful Suggestions" to shape your own suggestions to further what is currently your most important goals. For specific management of pain and other symptoms refer to comfort solution 6, "Finding Comfort," and comfort solution 8, "Adjusting Body Functions and Symptoms to Your Advantage;" in particular, see "Create an image of normal functioning" and/or "Create an image of healing."

Move your legs around

If your recovery includes bed rest, you need to prevent blood clots from forming in your legs. If you have to remain in bed for extended time periods keep moving your legs on a schedule (unless, of course, there is a medical reason not to do so). For example, while awake, every hour on the hour do toe lifts or press your toes against the footboard for five minutes; or if you watch TV, do so at every commercial break. The goal is to contract the calf muscles, which will help propel blood up from the legs so that it doesn't stay too long in one place, which would increase the risk of clotting. If you are at home, watch for these signs of blood clots: your leg becomes either swollen, abnormally hot, discolored, and/or superficial veins suddenly become much more prominent than before. If these symptoms occur, it is important to get medical help without delay.

Keep breathing deeply

Remind yourself on and off to consciously take deep breaths to keep your lungs fully inflated. If you had surgery and were given an incentive spirometer in the hospital, make sure you understand how to use it before taking it home—and use it faithfully until you are fully recovered and up and about again.

Guard against unhelpful suggestions

If your symptoms seen to be lingering, ask yourself if prior to your treatment someone may have implanted some negative ideas into your subconscious such as, "Oh you just have to live with the pain." The subconscious mind may have interpreted that statement as you need pain to live—therefore, if the pain leaves, there will be no life. Reflect on whether such statements happened and reframe the sentiment by making suggestions about your having a healthful and enjoyable future. Start imaging all the things you will be able to do with enjoyment and visualize yourself full of life and energy. Clearly imagine how you will look, how you will feel, and what you will do when healed.

Don't tough it out

Keep in mind that you don't have to prove anything to yourself or anybody else. There may be times where you may need to take a painkiller to get you over the initial recovery stages after surgery or dentistry. When that is the case, take the medication and take it early on. Don't wait until your tolerance has maxed out.

Give yourself a break

Overcome the urge to get all of the tasks that accumulated prior to your treatment taken care of in record time. Give your body enough rest to recover, but do get back into a healthy daily routine as soon as possible.

RELAXATION TECHNIQUES & SELF-HYPNOSIS

CHAPTER 15
Using Safe Non-Drug Comfort Solutions

Medical encounter stress can begin at first awareness of a health-related issue and continue right through diagnostic and treatment procedures. In addition to dealing with your specific health concern, you may have to make personal decisions with long-reaching ramifications. You want to do the right thing. You want relief and you want to keep your mind sharp and in control. Anti-anxiety drugs and pain killers are sometimes appropriate to give you the first, but to do so they all too often inherently force you to sacrifice the second. To get relief and keep control, you need a non-drug solution or at the least one that allows you to manage with a minimum of drugs—and drug side effects.

The quickest, ever-ready helpful choices are relaxation techniques. Many versions, such as relaxation breathing, are popular self-help solutions. They are easy to learn, discrete, and can be very effective in a number of situations. For step-by-step directions, see comfort solution 1, "Relaxation Breathing Technique."

For deeper comfort, especially in the more stressful situations, the best non-drug solution that can be accessed easily and quickly and can be done in any environment is *self-hypnosis*— a state of focused concentration and enhanced resourcefulness. Lack of information, misinformation, and exposure to long ago disproved myths about self-hypnosis have for too many years kept patients from this natural, safe, immediate approach to comfort.

Facts about Self-Hypnosis

It's not meditation. An important distinction between self-hypnotic and purely meditative practices is the focus on outcome. In hypnosis, mind and body become focused on a desired outcome and/or dealing with a presenting problem either by converting it into something manageable or by diverting thoughts actively to a more pleasant and empowering experience. Meditation, on the other hand, is typically performed for the sake of itself, and any resulting positive outcomes that occur are considered a nonspecific side effect. An exercise analogy for meditation is working out on a treadmill without a particular goal; the hypnotic counterpart is picking an exercise regimen geared towards getting in shape, completing a marathon, losing weight, feeling better, or any other specific desire.

It's not sleep. Self-hypnosis is not a state of sleepiness; the brain is actually working very actively during the hypnotic state. This state is quite natural, and it is likely that you are familiar with it. If you have ever been so completely absorbed in an activity (surfing the web, reading a book that you "just can't put down," or watching a spellbinding movie) that you noticed neither the passing of time nor what was going on around you, then you have already experienced the state of mind of self-hypnosis.

You cannot be forced into it. Nobody can make you get absorbed in a movie or book that you find boring. What's more, even if you like a book or movie nobody can make you get absorbed in it on command if you don't want to at this moment or have other priorities on your mind. Your control in those situations mirrors the control retained by a subject formally guided to enter self-hypnosis which cannot take place without the subject's willingness and cooperation.

You stay in control. All hypnosis is basically self-hypnosis. The subject remains in control and nobody can hypnotize anyone against his or her will. For example, nobody can make you cluck

Guided Self-Hypnosis:
The Comfort Talk® Experience

The keys to making self-hypnosis work for you are first to unlock your inner resources, and second, to focus those resources in a way that can enhance your medical experience and improve your overall medical outcome.

The strategies and step-by-step techniques for personal use presented in this book, *Managing Your Medical Experience*, grew from author Elvira Lang, MD's extensive research and her implementation in major medical centers of Comfort Talk® Training—a training system that provides medical staff with the knowledge and skills needed to help patients reframe their medical experience. The supporting structure of Comfort Talk® Training is *guided* self-hypnosis. Essentially the strategies are the same as those of self-hypnosis; in both the subject (patient) responds to suggestions to positively affect his or her current perception of sensations, emotions, and thoughts. The difference is that self-hypnosis, although it can incorporate written or audio learning guides, is essentially self-directed and self-initiated, while in guided self-hypnosis the subject (patient) is encouraged and guided by medical personal. Medical facility personnel throughout the US and elsewhere are being taught the Comfort Talk® guided self-hypnosis techniques to help patients help themselves to lessen or eliminate their need for painkillers, anxiety medicine, and other sedation drugs.

Honing skills in self-hypnosis can prepare you to make the most of the Comfort Talk® option where it is offered to patients. If your medical facility personnel have not yet been trained in Comfort Talk®, this book can give you the power to help yourself to create a safe, comfortable place that will always be there for you—even through a medical test or procedure. For more information about Comfort Talk® go to www.hypnalgesics.com.

like a chicken if you don't want to or would not find it fun to do so in the setting. Stage hypnotists very skillfully and carefully select their participants from the audience to assure their willingness and ability to act according to suggestions. Even in this setting, people will not do things they would find repugnant outside of the hypnotic experience.

It's natural. Self-hypnosis falls on a spectrum that also encompasses other naturally occurring experiences such as day dreaming, being on "auto-pilot," being lost in thought, praying, losing oneself in practicing yoga, zoning out during a run, and so forth. As some of these examples indicate, one doesn't even need to have the eyes closed or be inactive. The common denominator of these experiences is being in a *trance:* an altered state of consciousness with the focus directed inward or on a specific task, as well as experiencing decreased awareness of what is happening peripheral to that focus of attention. Self-hypnosis has the additional element of using trance towards a goal, in this context of helping yourself.

Elements of Self-Hypnosis

Essentially, self-hypnosis has several elements including:

- **Induction:** a formal procedure that gets the self-hypnosis session started. It can be a defined sequence of breaths or eye movements, counting of numbers, rhythmic movements, or some signal to enter trance that the subject gives him- or herself. Sometimes the induction can be as simple as asking oneself where one would rather be, invite oneself to think about where one always wants to go to.
- **Relaxation:** a process that closely follows and sometimes is part of the Induction. Some common examples of relaxation techniques include: Tightening and then releasing subsequent muscle groups from head to toe or vice versa. Thinking about letting tension

go with each breath out and taking in *strength* or *peace* with each breath in. Focusing on imagining a calming or healing light sent into muscles groups. Developing a sense of floating. Combining "floating" with a reach into "depth" such as "floating right through a chair or bed" or "floating deeper and deeper" can be particularly effective wordings even though in a non-hypnotic state these words seem illogical.

- **Positive imagery:** a technique in which subjects call to mind a pleasant scene where they would like to be instead of where they actually are at the moment. Sometimes people enjoy visiting exciting new settings, activities, or travel destinations they always wanted to explore. Other times people find soothing inside settings and activities that are familiar—sitting in a recliner at home reading a book, watching TV, or conducting routine work tasks.[1] The goal is mental immersion—the subject's body remains wherever it is, but his or her mind is free to bask in the image of him- or herself being in a pleasant, safe, comfortable place. To shape the perceived imagery, the subject employs all senses to "see," "feel," "hear," "smell," and "taste" the essence of the imagined scene. While imagery may imply pictures the term stands for any perceived experience element including those expressed in terms of sounds, feelings, tastes, or smells. People typically have a preferred sense—the particular sense they feel gives them the most profound connection with a scene, and in initiating imagery a person may give a bit more emphasis to his or her preferred sense. It is a good idea, however, to always include all the senses in the experience of positive imagery.
- **Anchoring:** the implicit association of a specific behavior or signal with a desirable state of mind so that it can later be used as a stimulus to bring the subject quickly back to this desirable state of mind.

- **Suggestions:** prompts to achieve the session's goals, which may reinforce positive feelings or reframe distressing thoughts.
- **Post-hypnotic suggestions:** suggestions that are intended to be followed beyond the end of the self-hypnosis session and be retained even after the subject becomes fully aware again.
- **Reorientation:** a formal procedure that returns the subject back to his or her natural state of awareness and alertness.

Because just entering a medical facility elicits a trance that aids in being focused on keeping oneself safe, one typically listens very carefully to every word that is said and is very attuned to surrounding noises,[2] we must add two obligatory elements to formal medical self-hypnosis:

- **Immunization against negative suggestions:** instructs the subject to accept only helpful suggestions and to ignore unhelpful ones. This element is necessary due to the unfortunately common incidents of medical staff inadvertently making statements that can be interpreted as negative, and given options of interpretation, the subconscious mind chooses the most literal negative interpretation possible.[3]
- **Immunization against noises:** instructs the subject to use noises in the room only to enhance his or her experience. This is necessary because medical facilities and some medical equipment are noisy enough to create stress.

For step-by-step directions for beginning to practice self-hypnosis see comfort solution 2, "Getting Started with Self-Hypnosis: the Basic Script."

Can Everyone Experience Self-Hypnosis?

The ability to enter self-hypnosis varies among people[4] and follows a bell-shaped curve.[5] About 10% of the population are highly hypnotizable enough that they can be guided through open surgery without medication. The good news is that everyone, even less or low hypnotizable individuals, can benefit from self-hypnosis in the medical encounter and experience greater comfort with it.[6] The level of hypnotizability or ability to get fully absorbed in imagined content provides some self-regulation in that context. Very anxious patients, who tend to be more hypnotizable,[7] are quite adept at imagining the "bad"—that is why they are anxious—but that also means that their mind is also very good at imaging the "good" when guided appropriately. Those on the low end of the spectrum who have a harder time entering self-hypnosis also tend to not imagine all possible calamities that cause the fears and anxieties of people with more vivid imaginations. All they may need are some simple relaxing and/or distracting instructions.

CHAPTER 16
Staying Comfortably Alert with Eyes-Open Self-Hypnosis

The half hour or so just before you will be talking to the doctor or brought into the treatment room or the surgical suite might seem an ideal time to close your eyes and practice your relaxation techniques and calm yourself. From a personal needs standpoint, it may be ideal to close your eyes and "let go," but your ability to remain focused during this critical time will impact the quality and quantity of the exchange of information between you and your healthcare professional, and may influence whether or not any outstanding issues get resolved before the procedure gets underway. Fortunately, you don't have to choose between self-hypnosis and eyes-open alertness. You can have both.

Eyes-Open Alert State vs. Eyes-Closed Drowsy State Self-Hypnosis

Hypnosis has long been associated with closed eyes and a detached state. Dr. James Braid, who introduced *hypnosis* in his 1843 book *Neurypnology,* derived the term from *Hypnos,* the Greek word for sleep.[1] However, *hypnosis* does not imply being sleepy or unable to converse. People tend to naturally enter a quasi-hypnotic state when injured or sufficiently stressed. A common example is the football player who can finish the game despite injury and only afterwards feels pain. Even Dr. Braid came to acknowledge that sleep was not an essential ingredient of hypnotism.[2] Children, guided by pediatric hypnotherapists are prime examples of effective open-eye hypnosis. Children easily experience a hypnotic state with their eyes open and even while moving around and playing out their imagined scenarios—playing pretend is one of their natural past times. For young children eyes-open hypnosis is actually the preferred approach.[3]

Dr. Wesley Raymond Wells, a professor at Syracuse University, was the first to put waking hypnosis to the test in an educational setting.[4] In class demonstrations he was able to show awake eyes-open hypnosis to be equally as powerful as "sleeping," eyes-closed techniques. Dr. Wells also suggested that the step to effective self-hypnosis was shorter with awake (eyes-open) hypnosis than it was with traditional eyes-closed hypnosis. Even when planning an eyes-closed hypnosis, Dr. Wells would first start with eyes-open induction.

Dr. David Wark, a psychologist at the University of Minnesota, has further refined eyes-open alert hypnosis in work with students who wanted to improve their levels of attention and participation during lectures and their retention of essential information, particularly for upcoming examinations.[5, 6] Research experiments with students demonstrate that subjects can remain self-hypnotized and give themselves self-suggestions with their eyes open and while walking, talking, or engaging in other activities. Additionally, and above all, they can experience therapeutic suggestions at the time and place where the problem occurs.[7] These demonstrated abilities make waking hypnosis particularly useful for the characteristically busy pre-op waiting time.

Eyes-open alert self-hypnosis uses successive elements of muscle tension and relaxation, associating in-breathing with a physical sensation and the feelings of strength and confidence; and out-breathing with relaxation. Because of its simplicity and proven track record of the approach that Dr. David Wark has perfected, my team chose that approach and adapted it over the years for use with patients awaiting or undergoing medical procedures and tests. The big advantage of eyes-open self-hypnosis is that patients can keep their eyes open and readily converse with healthcare professionals without interrupting their state of focused attention and the pursuit of their preset comfort goals. You can easily learn this approach and apply it whenever you need it.

Learning Eyes-Open Alert Self-Hypnosis

You can develop your skills in eyes-open alert self-hypnosis by first using it in low stress, outside-of-healthcare settings. To start, first set easy-to-evaluate goals. For example, you might suggest to yourself that you will closely concentrate when reading important information, that you will listen attentively to your conversation partner, that learning will be more interesting, and that you will retain more of what is important to you. Be sure to write down your suggestions. Next bring your skills to focus by suggesting that your use of self-hypnosis will become easier every time you practice. Write down that suggestion before you start, perhaps say: *I will find it easier and easier to enter a pleasant state of self-hypnosis.* Such exercises will help you develop your skills in executing eyes-open alert self-hypnosis so that you can easily access them as needed, regardless of the situation. You can practice and build your skill in five successive steps. For step-by-step directions for learning eyes-open alert self-hypnosis, see comfort solution 3, "Eyes-Open Alert Self-Hypnosis Steps."

Note that once you are familiar with the technique you may not need all steps for every occasion.

CHAPTER 17
Integrating Helpful Suggestions

Self-hypnosis is often used to enter a state of focused relaxation, but this state is not necessarily one of inactivity. Although self-hypnosis can relax and calm the mind, it can also be quite helpful in situations where you want to remain focused and physically active in order to pursue a goal. A common example of this active effort is when athletes enter a self-hypnotic state to bring themselves "in the zone" of confidence and high achievement performance.

Following the basic self-hypnosis script and instructions presented in comfort solution 2, "Getting Started with Self-Hypnosis: the Basic Script," and comfort solution 3, "Eyes-Open Alert Self-Hypnosis Steps," can transport you to a focused state that taps your inner resources for better outcome and performance. However, there may be times when you want to add elements to these basic scripts in order to accomplish a specific goal. In this book such additions are referred to as inserts; and the format for such goal-oriented inserts is the use of suggestions. Once in a self-hypnotic state, a person becomes more open to suggestions. In essence, it is because of this enhanced receptiveness to suggestions that I always recommend the inclusion of an immunization element to shield against anything that would be unhelpful to the subject while in a trance experience. Every induction should include the suggestion that you *will use all the sounds and noises to deepen your own experience and only listen to suggestions that are helpful for you and let the rest just pass by.* For further information on immunizations elements see chapter 15, "Using Safe Non-Drug Comfort Solutions." Also always make sure you reorient yourself to your natural state of awareness when the exercise is completed.

Structuring Suggestion Inserts

The content of an insert to the Basic Script is shaped by the specific goal being pursued. However, before you begin to formulate a suggestion aimed at helping you reach a specific goal, you need to consider the possibilities for structuring suggestion inserts.

Suggestions that link a desired reaction to a stimulus. If you have had or anticipate stress resulting from exposure to a specific event or type of situation, you may want to structure an insert suggestion that reframes the anticipated stimulus to trigger your desired reaction to it. This type of insert suggestion is best used when two criteria are met: First, the stimulus or event tends to produce a repeated, predictable, and unhelpful or disagreeable reaction; and second, a reframing reaction towards a more appropriate behavior will be helpful to you. For example, if you are nervous about a dental appointment, you might suggest that while you are in the dentist chair each time you hear the whir of the dental drill that sound will be a signal for you to go into even deeper relaxation. If you are vulnerable to excessive worrying and it starts with a knot in your stomach, you might suggest that each time you sense the knot forming, that sensation will be a signal to take five relaxing breaths—breathing in calm with each in-breath and letting go of worry with each breath out.

Suggestions that integrate external stimuli into a favorite imagery. If you include positive imagery (see Elements of Self-Hypnosis in chapter 15, "Using Safe Non-Drug Comfort Solutions") as part of your self-hypnosis experience, you may want to structure suggestions that integrate anticipated external stimuli into your imagery. Once you have "floated" to where you imagine yourself being or have started to associate with a place where you would rather be with all your senses, any new events in the physical environment can be integrated into the environment of your imagery. What's more, such suggestions may affect how a sensation is experienced. For example, if you imagine you are relaxing in the sunshine in a comfortable lounge chair in a wonderful vacation spot, and a real-world nurse or technician begins to rub cold disinfecting solution on your skin, you could imagine that the solution is a soothing sunscreen of welcome coolness protecting you from too much sun. Another common stimulus in medical settings is noise. Fortunately, noises are particularly well suited to support imagery, and just as you might choose to perceive cold disinfectant as a soothing sunscreen, you can incorporate surrounding noise into a natural element of your imagery. Alternatively you can use external stimuli to lead you into an imagery scenario you enjoy. For example, if you are a music lover, the sound of an MRI machine may remind you of the click of a metronome or the beat of a drum, either of which can be your free ticket to a front row seat at a concert of your musical preference choice.

Suggestions that link a feeling of the moment to an anchor. In self-hypnosis, an anchor is a reminder signal that can help you quickly return to a desired feeling—perhaps calm or comfortable—or to a state of mind—perhaps confident or focused—that you experienced while in self-hypnosis. An anchor can be a color, a sound, or just an easy action such as rubbing your thumb and forefinger together or curling your toes. You "set" your anchor when you are "experiencing" the desired feeling or emotion while you are in a self hypnotic state. Doing so at the moment of experience allows you to use the anchor to instantly retrieve that same sentiment whenever you need it. Guidelines for choosing and setting anchors are given below. Also see comfort solution 4, "Structuring Self-Hypnosis to Strengthen Self-Confidence."

Suggestions for implementation after the self-hypnosis session. *Posthypnotic suggestions* are suggestions that propose certain behaviors that you will perform after you re-emerge from the self-hypnotic state. These behaviors may or may not be tied to a signal that cues the action. Posthypnotic suggestions can aid healing, and can help with any other helpful behavior. For example, a posthypnotic suggestion cued to eating could help you to remember to take smaller bites and be sensitive to signals of satiety while enjoying every bite as a gourmet would.

Suggestions for Eyes-Open Alert Self-Hypnosis. These suggestions are meant for active participation within your immediate environment while experiencing self-hypnosis. Dr. David Wark did the original application of eyes-open self-hypnosis to students studying for upcoming tests. The students were able to remaining alert, take in information effortless, and easily retrieve it when needed for the test.[1, 2] The same process can be applied to other contexts. For example, if you are at the doctor's office, your suggestion might be, "I will remain calm, collected, and assertive until I have obtained all the information I need that is helpful for me." This type of suggestions will be highly personal; you can substitute any qualities you want to achieve and designate any context that is helpful for you. To construct suggestions for eyes-open self-hypnosis, use the same guidelines given for constructing closed-eye self-hypnosis suggestions.

Constructing Suggestion Inserts

Examples of suggestions relevant to various goals appear ready made in comfort solutions: 4, "Structuring Self-Hypnosis to Strengthen Self-Confidence," 5, "Using All Sounds to Aid Relaxation," 6, "Finding Comfort," and 7, "Taming Anxiety and Worries." You can also devise your own suggestions to exactly suit your needs. To get maximal effect from your suggestions, it's best to write your suggestions down and refine them before use. To construct effective suggestion, you need to first become familiar with hynoidal language, which you will need to use to phrase suggestions that will be optimally effective. Use the following approach:[3]

- **Phrase suggestions positively not negatively.** Because the subconscious mind remembers what is said even when a disclaimer is used, a negative suggestion would be counter productive. A classic example is to tell yourself NOT to think of pink elephants. Once you say the statement, it is difficult to think of anything other than a pink elephant. Similarly, you do not want to suggest to yourself, "I will NOT feel dread when in the pre-op area," because your subconscious mind will ignore the *not* and focus on the *feel dread when in the pre-op area*. The solution is to word the suggestion in a positive statement that tells what you WOULD like to feel. In this context, you might say "I will find it interesting to see first-hand the inner workings of a real hospital pre-op area, which many people can see only on TV or the movies. This will be so much better than Hollywood."

- **Be permissive and flexible.** Avoid suggestions for absolute and immediate success such as "I will be completely relaxed from now on all the time," or "I will never get angry again." Such wishful thinking can set a person up for failure and loss of confidence in the whole process. Instead, suggest a gradual progress with an open time frame such as "Soon I will find it easier and easier to relax," or "Gradually I will feel more and more in control in how I respond to whatever happens and find solutions that are most helpful for me."

- **Choose an appropriate anchor.** When you choose an anchor to elicit a feeling or action, it can be an external event or internal stimulus in form of a sight, sound, feeling, smell, or taste that you then link with a desirable outcome. With regard to external stimuli, you may be bound to what happens during a medical procedure. For example, you might insert the suggestion that, "each time the instrument touches my skin, that touch will be a signal for the area to develop even greater numbness."

When it comes to a signal you want to give yourself, it is best to bring yourself in your mind to a scenario that elicits the desired feeling and within that scenario choose a signal that speaks most to you in sensory terms and/or one that you want to evoke a certain reaction. If you are someone who likes to think in images, your anchor signal could be a color or image; if your experience is more framed by what you hear, your signal could be a sound or song you can think of or reproduce. If you tend to use words in your daily life that imply feelings, movements, and doing things, you could choose a feeling or movement—such as rubbing your thumb and fore finger together—as an anchor signal to bring you closer to your desired outcome. If tastes and smells are high on your list of what creates a full experience for you, taste or smell would be the anchor signal of choice. Thus, an anchoring signal is a ticket to return immediately into the feelings you experienced while in your referred scenario. You can go back there any time you wish just by thinking of your anchor signal—think of your anchor color or look at an item of that color; whistle your anchor song in you head, do a movement you associate with your anchor, or think of the smell or taste you have designated as your anchor signal.

- **Be very specific.** Instead of suggesting, "I will not feel anything and be numb," it is better to suggest, "I will feel numbness only where it needs to be numb, and only for as long it is helpful to be numb."

- **Keep suggestions short and write them out.** Write out precise, cogent, unambiguous suggestion inserts.

- **Implement them at the most effective time.** Suggestion inserts are most effective if you introduce them *after* your formal induction and *before* you are fully reoriented.

If you have time to practice adding inserts to the Basic Script before your medical encounter, do so. Practice will help you move smoothly through the process. You may want to begin with those suggestions in comfort solutions 4-7 that interest you or are pertinent right this moment. This practice will help you to better understand hypnotic phrasing and the process of using inserts to personalize the Basic Script. If the examples provided fall short of your needs, use the above guidelines to construct your own suggestions—and practice using them.

COMFORT SOLUTIONS FOR FAST RELIEF

Comfort Solutions are relaxation and self-hypnosis scripts, which you can follow to utilize your mind's natural ability to bring you the comfort you want by—depending on your need—overcoming pain, reducing stress, calming anxiety, or bolstering your self-confidence. Comfort solutions are structured so that you can enjoy immediate, general relief from the basic scripts, yet always have the option of personalizing a script. I will show you how with just a few quick additions, you can refine the script focus to conquer your specific challenges.

Still another option for fast relief is to utilize the Comfort Talk® downloadable app, which you can order directly from the Apple App Store or through the Hypnalgesics website at www.hypnalgesics.com/pages/pr.MyComfortTalkApp.html.

CAUTION: *While you are engaged in using the scripts or listening to the app, your attention will shift away from your external surroundings and the daily task at hand toward a more inward focus. Thus, you should not engage in this practice while driving, operating machinery, performing or tasks that requires your full attention to it or the surrounding environment.*

All comfort solutions are easy to understand and use, but do vary in complexity. The fastest and simplest approach to comfort is comfort solution 1: "Relaxation Breathing Technique," which is introduced in chapter 1, "Scheduling a Test; Waiting for Results." Although each of the comfort solutions is introduced in a book chapter, *Managing Your Medical Experience* is structured so that you can get right to the information you want/need. One option is to read through the chapters, pausing to investigate each comfort solution as it is introduced. However, Part II of the book—chapters 15, 16, and 17 together with the comfort solutions—is a self-contained tutorial providing all the information you need to bring yourself fast comfort through self-hypnosis.

Although the comfort solutions are related, each can stand-alone. Each comfort solution includes an alternative short introduction and reorientation paragraph. Also included is a framework so that even when you choose to personalize a script, you will always include the critical elements.

Comfort Solution	Topic focus	Related Chapters
1. Relaxation Breathing Technique	Breathing techniques for relaxation	1, 2
2. Getting Started with Self-Hypnosis: the Basic Script	Introduction to self-hypnosis: basic steps	15
3. Eyes-Open Alert Self-Hypnosis Steps	Keeping eyes open and staying alert during self-hypnosis	16
4. Structuring Self-Hypnosis to Strengthen Self-Confidence	How to boost self-confidence	6, 17
5. Using All Sounds to Aid Relaxation	How to cope with surrounding noise	9, 17
6. Finding Comfort	How to manage pain	11, 17
7. Taming Anxiety and Worries	How to manage anxiety	12, 17
8. Adjusting Body Functions and Symptoms to Your Advantage	How to affect medical symptoms	11, 13, 14, 17
9. Suggestions for Healing and Recovery	How to structure post-hypnotic suggestions	14, 17

Comfort Solution 1
Relaxation Breathing Technique

Also see chapter 1, "Scheduling a Test; Waiting for Results,"
and chapter 2, "Waiting for a Test or Treatment."

Best is to practice relaxation breathing a few times a day. You can just start with a few breaths and then expand as needed or as time permits. Relaxation breathing can also help you make the most out of a short break during the day and help you fall asleep at night. It is also a good preparation for self-hypnotic relaxation techniques.

Simple relaxation breathing

The following mind-body exercise can be done without preparation; you can do it anywhere—lying in bed, sitting, standing, walking, at home, at work, in the grocery store, and in the doctor's office. Just take a moment to focus on your breath, and:

- with each breath you take in think: "strength,"
- with each breath you breathe out think: "calm."

You may notice how even after just a few breaths you let more and more tension out of your body and start to feel calmer.

Breathing away unhelpful thoughts

If you want to work more on deeper relaxation or work on releasing specific anxieties, intruding thoughts, or worries, you can choose alternative wording, but then you should observe the precautions of not engaging in the practice when having to pay close attention to external tasks at hand.

For this alternative exercise, focus on your breath, and:

- With each breath you take in, focus on taking in strength, and

- with each breath out, focus on breathing out anything that is not helpful for you (anxiety, stress, tension, worries, or whatever bothers you).

- You may even feel how you grow taller with every breath you take in and your lungs filling with cleansing air and how with each breath out all the negative and unhelpful emotions and sensations just float away. Alternatively you can focus on blowing them actively out, perhaps even right through the skin. The latter works also well when what is bothering has a physical element— then you blow the bothering sensation right through the spot where you feel it.

Belly breathing

If you are lying down and don't have any special issues to address and just want to relax there is one more alternative:

You can close your eyes and place your hand on your belly, and take belly breath in and out, gently and regularly, just feeling the pro and fro of your belly lifting up and down. You can even imagine your rising and falling belly to be a beautiful balloon of your color of choice becoming larger and smaller with each breath in and out.

Comfort Solution 2
Getting Started with Self-Hypnosis: the Basic Script

Also see chapter 15, "Using Safe Non-Drug Comfort Solutions."

The following strategies introduce you to the practice of self-hypnosis with a short session as a first step toward becoming relaxed and ready for your medical encounter. This session uses the *Basic Script,* an adaptation of the *Study Script,* which was developed and refined for use in the clinical trials that I oversaw. Subsequently, the script was put into clinical use with thousands of patients having medical procedures and tests.

CAUTION: *While engaging in self-hypnotic relaxation do not drive or perform activities that requires your direct attention.*

Step 1: Familiarize yourself with the elements and language of self-hypnosis.

To become familiar with the language and elements of self-hypnosis, please first read through the Basic Script that follows. At this stage don't attempt yet to enter a trance. After you read it through once, use the bulleted list of the elements of self-hypnosis that appears in chapter 16, "Using Safe Non-Drug Comfort Solutions" as a resource to help you identify the self-hypnosis elements addressed in each sentence of the Basic Script. Noise in the environment doesn't matter. If it is quiet around you that is fine, but this script also holds up quite well in noisy environments.

NOTE: The following script and other Comfort Solution scripts are constructed on the assumption that someone will read the script aloud to the self-hypnosis subject. The reader may be another voice or you may make a recording of yourself reading the script to playback for your own use. In the script, the subject is addressed as *you*. If you prefer to address yourself in the first person, simply substitute the appropriate personal pronoun *(I, me, my, myself)* for each use of *you, your, yourself* in the script. To aid substitution, pronouns appear in Italic print.

The Basic Script

If *you* hear sounds or noises in the room, just use these to deepen *your* own experience. And use only useful suggestions that are helpful for *you* and let the rest just go by.

There are a lot of ways to relax, but here is one simple way.

On *one*, do one thing: look up (pick any spot *you* like on the ceiling)

On *two*, do *two* things: slowly close *your* eyes and take a deep breath in.

On *three*, do *three* things: breathe out, relax the eyes, and let *your* body float.

… Just imagine *your* whole body floating, floating right through the table (or bed, or chair *you* are on), with each breath deeper and easier. And with each breath *you* breathe in, take in strength, and with each breath *you* breathe out, think calm. Right now imagine that *you* are floating somewhere safe and comfortable, in a bath, a lake, a hot tub, or just floating in space, with each breath deeper and easier.

… Just notice how with each breath *you* let a little more tension out of *your* body as *you* let *your* whole body float, safe and comfortable; each breath deeper and easier.

… Good, remaining in this state of concentration and with *your* eyes closed, reflect on how *your* body is feeling right now. Where do *you* imagine *yourself* being? Just enjoy for *yourself* what it is like? Can *you* smell the air? Can *you* see what is around *you*? …

… Good.

… Now this is *your* safe and pleasant place to be and *you* can use it in a sense to play a trick on whatever happens around *you* now or during *your* medical procedure and *you* can always return to it. *Your* body has to be here, but *you* don't. So just spend *your* time being somewhere *you* would rather be.

Option. At this point you may insert helpful suggestions targeted to your specific goals. To inserts your own suggestion, see chapter 17, "Integrating Helpful Suggestions." For prepared suggestions for specific topics, see comfort solutions 5 through 9.

...When *you* are ready to leave this state of focused concentration *you* can start counting backwards from three to one. On *three* get ready, on *two* with *your* eyes closed roll up *your* eyes, and on *one* let *your* eyes open and take a deep breath and let it out. That will be the end of the formal exercise, but when *you* come out of it, *you* will still have the feeling of comfort that *you* felt during it and be proud to have learned how *you* can help *yourself*.

Step 2: Set up your delivery system.

As explained above, language is such an important component of the self-hypnotic process that it is best at first to follow along a script as written. It is also helpful to hear the script. You can read the script; speak it out loud, or record yourself reading the script on your phone or recorder. If you prefer to hear a different voice, you might have someone else read it or even record the script for you. Still another option is to utilize the My Comfort Talk® downloadable app. You can download it directly from the Apple App Store or go to the Hypnalgesics website at www.hypnalgesics. com/pages/pr.MyComfortTalkApp.html.

Step 3: Put self-hypnotic relaxation into practice.

Once you have listened a few times to your audio recording and practiced an "eye roll" induction, you will find it easier and easier to do it on your own even at a moment's notice and without any props or tapes. Sometimes an eye roll is all that is needed to get you into a state of relaxation and the reorientation sentences (reversed eye roll) to get you back to your natural state of awareness.

Regardless how much you abbreviate, and even when you are by yourself and everything promises to be perfectly quiet and without interruptions, make a habit to always tell yourself: "I will use all the sounds and noises in the room to deepen my own experience and I will listen only to suggestions that are helpful for me." These also should be the very first suggestions you give yourself whenever entering a medical space or conversation.

Step 4: Personalize your experience.

You can easily alter the Basic Script to make it suit your situation more precisely by adding inserts to the script. Inserts are suggestions that enforce a specific goal. For guidance on writing self-hypnosis script inserts to personalize your experience, see chapter 17, "Integrating Helpful Suggestions." You will also find many ideas in comfort solutions 5 through 9.

Comfort Solution 3
Eyes-Open Alert Self-Hypnosis Steps

Also see chapter 16, "Staying Comfortably Alert with Eyes-Open Self-Hypnosis."

You can practice and build your skill in eyes-open alert self-hypnosis by following the five steps described below. Get comfortable before you begin, ideally with your feet on a firm surface. You can sit in a chair with your feet on the floor, or if you are in a hospital bed or gurney sit with your legs bent and your feet planted on the mattress, if you can.

Step 1: Take a deep breath.

To begin, gently take a deep breath, hold it for a moment, and then gently breathe out. It doesn't need to be an enormous breath, just a comfortable breath. Notice how with your inhalation you become taller, your neck extending gently upwards and slightly backwards, your shoulders rising and with the exhalation your rib cage becomes smaller, your shoulders move down, and your head moves slightly forward and down. Once you feel the rise and fall with inspiration and expiration you can go to step 2. Until then, practice a bit more with step 1.

Step 2: Hold your next breath.

Take another breath and hold it   and while you hold your breath, push down on your feet and slightly tense your feet, ankles, calves, and thighs. Now, exhale. You may notice that the sensation of growing taller with the in-breath and looser with the out-breath is even more noticeable than in step 1. You can repeat step 2 as often as you like until you become fully aware of the sensations; then move on to step 3.

Step 3: Tighten your muscles

Take another breath in and tighten every muscle in your body from your toes to your head—becoming really really tall. Feel the tension. Then slowly exhale and let your whole body relax.

Option. Practice steps 1-3 for warm-up as often as you like until you develop a sense for the changes that occur with each breath. When you are ready, move to step 4: eye fixation induction. An *induction* is the ritual or signal you give your mind to enter a state of focused attention and prepare to receive suggestions, which you can initiate. Open-eye induction basically involves doing steps 1-3 in sequence while you do step 4, which is to focus on one any spot on the wall or in the distance that you like.

Step 4: Eye fixation

Make yourself comfortable, then pick a "spot" in front of you at eye level or slightly higher—a painting, light switch, wall-mounted equipment, irregularity or patterns on a wall, or anything in your line of sight that is not likely to be moved. Keep your eyes focused on your chosen spot while you take a breath in. Feel yourself grow tall as the air streams gently into your lungs; hold your breath for a moment, and then relax, breathing any tension out (step 1). With your next breath in, gently push your feet against the surface, tense your ankles, calves, and thighs; become tall, hold your breath, and breathe out (step 2). Keep your eyes focused on the spot as you take in another breath. As you become really tall, tense your entire body, hold your breath, and then breathe out— releasing all tension along with your breath (step 3). Keep focusing on your spot (step 4) as you keep breathing normally; taking in strength and clarity with each breath in; releasing any remaining tension with each breath out.

After you have done your three breaths; becoming tall and then relaxed (steps 1-3), and breathing calmly while keeping your eyes on the spot (step 4), notice if the spot changes color or shape in relationship to its surroundings. You may feel yourself go deeper and deeper into a state of self-hypnosis. You may feel yourself swaying or moving a little, and you may sense your focus shifting. You can engage in any pleasant scenario that comes to mind— a wonderful place, a gorgeous day, or just an imagined pleasant sense of floating somewhere safe and comfortable—whatever comes up; enjoy it with all your senses.

Option. At this point you may insert helpful suggestions targeted to your specific goals. To insert your own suggestion, see Chapter 17, "Integrating Helpful Suggestions." For prepared suggestions for specific topics, see comfort solutions 5 through 9.

NOTE: You are always in control and can re-alert yourself anytime if needed or desired. You can quickly come out of eyes-open alert self-hypnosis simply by blinking your eyes. Use blinking to re-alert yourself to your natural state of awareness any time you wish to do so. Notice how you feel after you re-alert yourself. Do you feel calmer or perhaps more energetic? You can also always quickly re-enter the eyes-open alert self-hypnosis state by performing the three breathing steps while focusing your eyes on a preferred spot.

Optional transitioning into Eyes-Closed Hypnosis

Your medical visit may be conducted and concluded all with eyes-open alert hypnosis, but if you are brought into a procedure room or are in a dentist chair and closing your eyes is an option, you can transition into eyes-closed hypnosis. You may already notice how your eyes want to close anyhow—so just allow them to close and engage in your own imagery, as you would do during any regular eyes closed self-hypnotic session.

Re-alerting yourself to end the session

At the end of your session, bring yourself to full awareness. You can formally end your state of self-hypnosis by blinking as discussed above or by counting backwards from three to one: At *three* look up, at *two* take in a deep breath, and at *one* breathe out and blink to become fully alert with your eyes wide open.

Comfort Solution 4
Structuring Self-Hypnosis to Strengthen Self-Confidence

Also see chapter 6, "Boosting Your Self-Confidence."

A very effective technique for calling upon and strengthening your self-confidence is to use self-hypnosis: First fully immerse yourself in a feeling of confidence and then to choose one element of the immersion experience as an *anchor*—a reminder of your feeling confident—that you can easily recall. Immersion can be easily achieved by using the Confidence Script below. When the script leads you to fully immerse yourself in a scenario in which you feel confident, enjoy the scene with all your senses—vision, hearing, smell, taste, and touch. You might find that one of your senses best represents the experience to you. If that is the case, use an object or action expressed by this favorite sense as an anchor you can call on to transport you back into your experience of feeling confident. For example, if you find that a color best represent the scenario you experienced while using to the Confidence Script, you can keep an object of that color at hand to help you re-enter that state of confidence. The object, which essentially operates as a "security blanket," could be a pen, a pair of socks—anything of that color; or you may just think of the color.

Perhaps, it wasn't a color but a sound that was elemental in your experience. If so, you may want to pick a melody or song to be your anchor. When you want to return to the experience of full confidence, just hum the tune—aloud or silently. If touch can best transport you back, you may enjoy giving yourself a reminder signal of your confidence immersion experience by rubbing your thumb and forefinger together or by curling your toes or by any other movement signal you prefer that you can apply anywhere without it being necessarily obvious to others.

Your anchor, your signal, is your ever-ready ticket back to that feeling of being in a self-confident state. When things are getting stressful, touch or think of your color, hum your song, or do your predetermined movement and look for the effect. You can also go through the Confidence Script again to relieve a state of self-confidence. Each time that you go through the script you continue building your confidence. You may be surprised how these sessions affect your daily life and behavior. The Confidence Script also works quite well when you want to fall asleep at night and all kind of thoughts are going through your mind. Going through the script encourages interesting and pleasant dreams.

CAUTION: *While engaging in self-hypnotic relaxation do not drive or perform activities that requires your direct attention.*

NOTE: The introduction and reorientation parts of the Confidence Script (marked by a gray line running alongside the text) are modeled on the Basic Script in comfort solution 2, "Getting Started with Self-Hypnosis: the Basic Script." The unmarked text sections in between are inserts specific for strengthening self-confidence.

In the script, the subject is addressed as you. If you prefer to address yourself in the first person, simply substitute the appropriate personal pronoun *(I, me, my, myself)* for each use of *you, your, yourself* in the script. To aid substitution, pronouns appear in Italic print.

Confidence Script

Ready to feel more confident and resourceful? Just use all the sounds and noises to deepen *your* own experience and use only suggestions that are helpful for *you.*

Then let's get started:

One: Look up

Two: breathe in and slowly close *your* eyes, and

Three: breathe out, relax *your* eyes and let *your* body float.

> ... Just imagine *your* whole body floating, with each breath deeper
> and easier. And with each breath *you* breathe in, take in strength,
> and with each breath *you* breathe out, think calm. Right now
> imagine that *you* are floating somewhere safe and comfortable, in
> a bath, a lake, a hot tub, or just floating in space, with each breath
> deeper and easier.

... Now, *you* can float to one of these "magical" moments when
everything just "clicks" and comes together perfectly. It may be a
private moment or a public achievement, when something came
true and through for *you* because *you* worked hard. *You* might
have persevered and succeeded, or something is just happening,
something good, something good just by itself. Or *you* may have
learned something and now it comes in handy in this amazing
way. *You* really can say, "Yes! This is it!" and *you* fully experience
the delight of this feeling. If *you* cannot think of such a personal
experience like that right now, imagine what it might be like to
have such an experience. Perhaps *you* have seen an experience
like that in a movie, or have heard a story about someone having
such an experience. Put *yourself* fully into that scenario.

... Good. Now float further down into this magical moment in
which everything just works out well. Enjoy this moment and
savor the sights and sounds; wrap the feelings of achievement and
delight around *you*.

... *You* might even notice a color that permeates the scene. If so,
you can make this "*your* color" and whenever—later in *your* work
and life—*you* wish to regain this wonderful state of accomplishment, confidence, and peace, *you* may just want to think of this
color. *You* may even want to keep at hand an object of "*your*" color
to remind *you* how to enter that state of self-assurance whenever
you need it, but just thinking of the color can be a signal in itself. Or
there may be a sound or song in the air that can be *your* reminder
of this moment, and just recalling this sound or song can transport
you back to this state of strength whenever *you* wish or need to.

128

... Alternatively, *you* can put thumb and forefinger together while immersed in the experience, and, hereafter, *you* can use this touching of the thumb and forefinger as a signal to bring to *you* this feeling of accomplishment, confidence, and peace that *you* are enjoying now. *You* can use one or more of these techniques whenever *you* desire or need to return to that confident state, even in the toughest of circumstances.

... One more thing, *your* unconscious mind has been going through a process of allowing itself to assimilate and organize all the information that *you* needed into a format that *your* conscious mind could easily use at any time. Although *you* may not be fully conscious of what *your* unconscious mind has processed, bring that information with *you* as *you* slowly float back above *yourself*.

> When *you* are ready to return to *your* natural state of awareness, slowly count backwards from three to one, as follows: On *three*, take a deep breath in. On *two*, let a breath out. On *one*, be fully awake, delighted, and proud to know how *you* can use *your* mind to relax, and how *you* can use *your* mind to help *yourself* and be effective.

Comfort Solution 5
Using All Sounds to Aid Relaxation

Also see chapter 9, "Tuning Out the Noise."

Some hospital noises, particularly those that are a fundamental part of treatment or imaging technology, cannot be silenced, but you can use those and all other sounds to your advantage. You can integrate sounds in the context of a formal self-hypnosis (see comfort solution 2, "Getting Started with Self-Hypnosis: the Basic Script," and chapter 15, "Using Safe Non-Drug Comfort Solutions") or address sounds directly—as a stand-alone approach. Because the mere act of participating in a medical encounter tends to place everyone into a natural hypnotic state, the suggestions below will work on their own or as part of a formal self-hypnosis script.

Sounds as an ally

As a safeguard, always give yourself a specific suggestions regarding noise at the beginning of your self-hypnosis induction or whenever you put foot in a medical facility: Say to yourself, "I will use all the sounds and noises as a signal to go into even deeper relaxation," or "I will use all the sound and noises to further deepen my own experience." And while you are at it add the next sentence "And I will only listen to suggestions that are helpful for me." These are the two most powerful sentences you can use in any medical encounter.

Sounds associated with unpleasant stimuli

Biopsy procedures often entail devices that make sounds: "Biopsy guns" (whoever came up with that negative suggestive expression!) thrust a sampling needle forward with a snapping sound;

vacuum pumps make their own distinct noise. In clinical practice, I learned to use these sounds to the patient's advantage. I always operate the equipment once outside the patient so that the patient could hear the associated sound. Upon making the sound, I simultaneously suggest that the patient use this intermittent sound as a signal to deepen even further his or her experience. And it really works! You can do the same for yourself. If sound goes along with an unpleasant stimulus, such as the sound of an instrument or machine that is part of a medical procedure, tell yourself, "Every time I hear this sound, I will relax even more."

Sounds that signal a painful stimulus

If you notice a sound just a moment before a painful stimulus affects your body, it becomes an alerting signal. Some examples are the clicking of a foot pedal, starting of a rotor, or other vibrations. You can use all of these sounds to deepen your relaxation. Tell yourself, "Every time I hear (the sound), it will be a signal to go deeper into relaxation," or "Every time I hear (the sound), it will be a signal for the area to develop even greater numbness," (if the procedure affects only a defined area) or "Every time I hear (the sound) it will be a signal to be strong, numb and courageous, and numb for as long and for where it need to be." The same principle can also be applied to other signals such as light flashes during laser treatment or the feeling of equipment touching you.

Continuous sounds

When you are experiencing sounds that are continuous for longer stretches of time, such as during an MRI scan, it is best to integrate that sound into the imagery that comes spontaneously to your mind when asking yourself where you would rather be. Then just consider what sounds may be associated with that imagery. Ideal are scenarios familiar to you and in which you can display mastery. For example, patients have associated the sound of the MRI machine with imagery of conducting a concert, riding a roller coasters, driving speed vehicles, listening to the old heating pipes at home clunking, or working with equipment, just to name a few. These choices are very individual and they will come up more or less by themselves and are experienced as soothing. It's your choice, and the best part is you can change imagery midstream. One patient who had been quite reluctant to undergoing an MRI scan initially decided to go on an imaginary trip to Disney Land during his scan which he enjoyed for a while. Then the thumps of the machine reminded him to the sound of a jackhammer— a tool he had used and enjoyed using. And that is what he did for the next 40 minutes – jack hammering. Our team has found that it is not uncommon for patients to choose activities that may seem mundane and not what would appear to an outsider as a pleasant activity of choice. What's important is it works for you.

Comfort Solution 6
Finding Comfort

Also see chapter 11, "Easing Pain."

Below are two self-hypnosis script options for easing pain. Option 1 is relatively generic and fast; Option 2 is a longer approach that uses the specific imagery of a floating stone with an additional reminder sentence (mantra).

CAUTION: *While engaging in self-hypnotic relaxation do not drive or perform activities that requires your direct attention.*

NOTE: In both options, the introduction and reorientation parts (marked by a gray line running alongside the text) are modeled on the Basic Script in comfort solution 2, "Getting Started with Self-Hypnosis: the Basic Script." The unmarked text sections in between accommodate inserts specific for pain management. You can use either option or even combine the middle parts.

In the script, the subject is addressed as *you*. If you prefer to address yourself in the first person, simply substitute the appropriate personal pronoun *(I, me, my, myself)* for each use of *you, your, yourself* in the script. To aid substitution, pronouns appear in Italic print.

Option 1: General comfort management

Use all the sounds and noises to deepen *your* own experience and use only suggestions that are helpful for *you*. Resting *your* head and body comfortably *you* may proceed:

On *one*, do one thing: look up (pick any spot *you* like on the ceiling)

On *two*, do *two* things: slowly close *your* eyes and take a deep breath in.

On *three*, do *three* things: breathe out, relax the eyes, and let *your* body float.

... Good. Just imagine *your* whole body floating, with each breath deeper and easier. And with each breath take in in strength, and with each breath out think "calm." Right now imagine that *you* are floating somewhere safe and comfortable, in a bath, a lake, a hot tub, or just floating in space, with each breath deeper and easier. Just notice how with each breath *you* let a little more tension out of *your* body as *you* let *your* whole body float, safe and comfortable; each breath deeper and easier. Good, now remaining in this state of concentration, focus on how *your* body is feeling right now. Where do *you* imagine *yourself* being? What is it like? Can *you* smell the air? Can *you* see what is around *you*? Good. Now this is *your* safe and pleasant place to be and *you* can use it in a sense to play a trick on whatever may happen and *you* can always return to it. *Your* body has to be here, but *you* don't. So just spend *your* time being somewhere *you* would rather be.

... Now, if there is some discomfort, and there may be some, there is no point in fighting it. *You* can admit it, but then transform that sensation. If *you* feel some discomfort, *you* might find it helpful to make that part of *your* body to feel warmer, as if *you* were in a bath. Or cooler—if that is more comfortable—as if *you* had ice or snow on that part of *your* body. This warmth and coolness becomes a protective filter between *you* and the pain.

... If *you* have any discomfort right now, imagine that *you* are applying a hot pack or that *you* are putting snow or ice on it and see what it feels like. Develop the sense of warm or cool or delicious tingling numbness to filter the hurt out of the pain. With each breath, breathe deeper and easier, *your* body is floating. Now, again with *your* eyes closed and remaining in the state of concentration, just note what *you* are feeling right now.

... If comfort has returned just keep imagining *yourself* being at *your* preferred place of safety where *you* enjoy being and where *you* felt relaxed and comfortable. What is it like now? What is the temperature? What do *you* see around you? If *you* wish *you* can add more coolness or more warmth to any area that might still bother *you* or make it lighter or make it heavier.

... *You* can also focus on sensations in another part of *your* body. *You* can rub *your* fingertips together and notice all of the delicate sensations in *your* fingertips and see how much *you* can observe about what it feels like to rub *your* thumb and forefingers together. Continue to focus on these sensations. And remember how *you* can take the hurt out of the pain.

... Just keep enjoying *yourself* in *your* place of delight with comfort and in a state of relaxation. And seconds can seems like minutes and minutes like hours when body and mind are at ease. And *you* can carry this feeling with *you* when *your* return to the here and now.

> When *you* are ready to formally leave this state of concentration *you* can do so by counting backwards from three to one. On *three*, get ready, on *two*, with *your* eyes closed roll up *your* eyes, and on *one*, let *your* eyes open and take a deep breath and let it out. That will be the end of the formal exercise, but when *you* come out of it, *you* will still have the feeling of peace and comfort that *you* felt during it.
>
> Ready, *three*, *two*, *one*.
>
> Take a deep breath, and feel refreshed and proud about knowing how to help *yourself* at any time to feel calm, strong, and resourceful.

Option 2: The Floating Stone

> Use all the sounds and noises to deepen *your* own experience and use only suggestions that are helpful for *you*.
>
> Resting *your* head and body comfortably *you* may proceed:
>
> On *one*, do one thing: look up (pick any spot *you* like on the ceiling)
>
> On *two*, do *two* things: slowly close *your* eyes and take a deep breath in.

> On *three*, do *three* things: breathe out, relax the eyes, and let *your* body float.
>
> ... Good. Just imagine *your* whole body floating, floating right through *your* chair or bed with each breath easier and deeper. Right now imagine that *you* are floating somewhere safe and comfortable, in a bath, a lake, a hot tub, or just floating in space, with each breath deeper and easier. Just notice how with each breath *you* let a little more tension out of *your* body as *you* let *your* whole body float, safe and comfortable; each breath deeper and easier. Where do *you* imagine *yourself* being? What is it like? Can *you* smell the air? Can *you* see what is around *you*? Now this is *your* safe and pleasant place to be and *you* can use it in a sense to play a trick on whatever may happen and *you* can always return to it. *Your* body has to be here, but *you* don't. So just spend *your* time being somewhere *you* would rather be.

... *You* may be on a beach or lake, walking down a solid path, or at home looking out the window, or just floating in space. Wherever *you* find *yourself* and enjoy *yourself* being, *you* can go there now.

... Perhaps *you* can see a child or someone on the shore of a calm clear lake about to skip a stone in the surface. And as the stone skips along on the surface of the water, it ripples away all anxiety, discomfort, fears, stresses, and strains. And *you* can feel, hear and see all discomfort floating away. Just as the stone is skipping over the glistening surface of the lake, with the beautiful colors of the sun breaking like in a prism, and all the beautiful colors and views that *you* might have ever seen and imagined.

... And as the stone ripples away, it comes to a place where it begins to float down—down to the first deep floor, way down to floor A. And just as the stone floats down, *you* float into a deeper state of relaxation safely and gently. And now while the stone floats down even deeper to the second deep floor, floor B, *you* can reach deeper levels of relaxation. *You* can test if *you* have arrived at floor B of relaxation. *You* can try to say the letter B but *you* cannot. And why bother.

... And while the stone is floating down even deeper into the water, it goes all the way down to the bottom of the lake, floor C, *you* can try to say the letter C, but no matter how hard *you* try, *you* cannot. And again why bother. And as *you* remain in *your* safe and pleasant place, *you* can notice how good it feels to relax like this and enjoy this wonderful deep relaxation all the way down, very deep, drifting and just as the stone, not feel a thing, just go with the flow. That's right. Resting on the bottom of the lake, just resting and going with the flow, the stone does not feel a thing.

... And *you* can say to *yourself* in *your* state of safe and secure floating: strong, numb, courageous, and safe—and numb only for where and for how long it need be. From now on this can be *your* mantra: strong, numb, courageous, and safe—and numb only for where and for how long it need be.

... And should *you* be preparing for a procedure or undergoing one, *you* can take all the stimuli as signals to go into even deeper relaxation and experience even greater numbness. This could be recurring sounds, or the flickering of lights, or bumps, or noticing *you* touching the equipment or it touching *you*—just use all the stimuli as signals to help *you* even further to enjoy *your* own experience of being strong, numb, courageous, and safe—and numb only for where and for how long it need be.

... And when this session or *your* procedure is completed and *you* are recovering perfectly. From now on anytime *you* might feel any discomfort *you* can go to the place *you* enjoy. All *you* have to do is close *your* eyes, breathe deeply, hold *your* thumb and forefinger together, and go to this wonderful place of security and comfort that *you* have just enjoyed. And isn't it nice to know that *you* can help *yourself*?

... And *you* can come back now, easily, gently and safely and as slowly or quickly, as *you* like. And when *you* are ready to come back *you* can begin to float up from floor C to floor B and then to floor A and when *you* reach floor A *you* are now in a light and waking state.

So now *you* can count *yourself* up from three to one and when *you* reach one *you* will be fully alert, fully awake, feeling better than *you* have in a long, long time from these few brief minutes of self-hypnosis, taking all the time *you* need. On *three* get ready, on *two* with *your* eyes still closed roll up *your* eyes, and on *one* let *your* eyes open and take a deep breath in and let it out.

Comfort Solution 7
Taming Anxieties and Worries

Also see chapter 12, "Soothing Anxiety."

Anxiety management typically consists of moving the bothersome feelings outside of your head and body so that they can be safely sent away or objectively observed and analyzed so you can design a concrete solution. Depending on the situation, taking some relaxation breaths as directed in comfort solution 1, "Relaxation Breathing Technique," may be all you need, or following a basic self-hypnotic induction as described in comfort solution 2, "Getting Started with Self-Hypnosis: the Basic Script," may suffice. Additionally, there are techniques in which your worries are set aside and carried away or your problems are isolated to help you generate solutions. The self-hypnosis script options below: The Red Balloon, Pile of Sand, and Split Screen are examples of these techniques.

CAUTION: *While engaging in self-hypnotic relaxation do not drive or perform activities that requires your direct attention.*

NOTE: In all options, the introduction and reorientation parts (marked by a gray line running alongside the text) are modeled on the Basic Script in comfort solution 2, "Getting Started with Self-Hypnosis: the Basic Script." The unmarked text sections in between accommodate inserts specific for anxiety management.

Option: The Red Balloon

Use all the sounds and noises to deepen *your* own experience and use only suggestions that are helpful for *you*.

Resting *your* head and body comfortably *you* may proceed:

On *one*, do *one* thing: look up (pick any spot *you* like on the ceiling)

On *two*, do *two* things: slowly close *your* eyes and take a deep breath in.

On *three*, do *three* things: breathe out, relax the eyes, and let *your* body float.

... Good. Just imagine *your* whole body floating, floating with each breath easier and deeper right through where *you* are resting. Right now imagine that *you* are floating somewhere safe and comfortable, in a bath, a lake, a hot tub, or just floating in space, with each breath deeper and easier. With each breath in, take in strength and with each breath out, think "calm" and let go of whatever there is to let go of. Just notice how with each breath *you* let a little more tension out of *your* body as *you* let *your* whole body float, safe and comfortable; each breath deeper and easier.

... Just remain in this state of concentration, focused on how *your* body is feeling right now. Where do *you* imagine *yourself* being? What is it like? Can *you* smell the air? Can *you* see what is around *you*? Good. Now this is *your* safe and pleasant place to be, and *you* can use it in a sense to play a trick on whatever may happen and *you* can always return to it.

... And while in this place where *you* enjoy the way *you* feel, *you* might imagine a valley lush with vegetation. Down in the valley *you* can see a large red balloon. As *you* walk toward the balloon, it appears bigger and bigger. Now *you* see that the balloon is attached to a large basket and that the basket is weighted down by large sand bags. In the basket is a large container.

... *You* can take the container out of the basket and fill it with *your* self-doubts, worries, fears, guilt, and discomforts. There is room

140

in the container for all *you* want to put in it. The more self-doubts and anxieties *you* put in the container, the more comfortable and confident *you* can become. Imagine filling the container. When *you* have filled the container as full as *you* wish with *your* self-doubts, worries, fears, guilt, and discomforts, take a deep satisfying breath. Feel calmer, more relaxed, and more confident.

... Now imagine placing the container back into the basket. Imagine the good feelings that doing this gives *you*. Now imagine *your* hands untying the ropes that hold the basket to the weights. As each rope is untied, a sandbag falls to the ground. As the sandbags fall, *you* have the power to let go, to release *yourself*, to enjoy life more. When the last bag falls, the basket begins to rise into the air.

... As the red balloon lifts, *you* can feel the burdens of self-doubt being lifted from *your* shoulders. As the balloon rises higher and higher, *you* feel a greater and greater distance from *your* self-doubts. Make this image as vivid and as detailed as *you* can. *You* can repeat and change the image as often as *you* like—now and also later when *you* return to *your* natural state of awareness. *You* can recreate this experience whenever *you* wish. When *you* imagine the color of the balloon, or the ropes holding the bags, or the container in the basket, it can be a signal for *your* self-doubts to flee. *You* can always carry with *you* the capacity to change in a positive way and bring relief to *yourself*.

> When *you* are ready to formally leave this state of concentration *you* can do so by counting backwards from three to one. On *three*, get ready, on *two*, with *your* eyes closed roll up *your* eyes, and on *one*, let *your* eyes open and take a deep breath and let it out. That will be the end of the formal exercise, but when *you* come out of it, *you* will still have the feeling of peace and comfort that *you* felt during it.
>
> Ready, *three*, *two*, *one*.
>
> Take a deep breath, and feel refreshed and proud about knowing how to help *yourself* at any time to feel calm, strong, and resourceful.

Option: Pile of Sand

Use all the sounds and noises to deepen *your* own experience and use only suggestions that are helpful for *you*. Resting *your* head and body comfortably *you* may proceed:

On *one*, do *one* thing: look up (pick any spot *you* like on the ceiling)

On *two*, do *two* things: slowly close *your* eyes and take a deep breath in.

On *three*, do *three* things: breathe out, relax the eyes, and let *your* body float.

... Good. Just imagine *your* whole body floating, floating with each breath easier and deeper right through where *you* are resting. Right now imagine that *you* are floating somewhere safe and comfortable, in a bath, a lake, a hot tub, or just floating in space, with each breath deeper and easier. With each breath in, take in strength and with each breath out, think "calm" and let go whatever there is to let go of. Just notice how with each breath *you* let a little more tension out of *your* body as *you* let *your* whole body float, safe and comfortable; each breath deeper and easier.

... Just remain in this state of concentration, focus on how *your* body is feeling right now. Where do *you* imagine *yourself* being? What is it like? Can *you* smell the air? Can *you* see what is around *you*? Good. Now this is *your* safe and pleasant place to be and *you* can use it in a sense to play a trick on whatever may happen and *you* can always return to it.

... *You* might enjoy imagining *yourself* building a pile of sand on a beach. Take all *your* worries, anxieties, and all feelings that are not helpful and just pile them up, build them into a huge pile, like a pile of sand. And have the pile grow bigger and bigger, just throw everything on it, everything that comes to mind, pile it on with abandon, the more the better—just throw it all on, just really build it up. Make it as high as it needs to be. That's right. Take all the time *you* need and get it all piled up. Then take a few breaths and start thinking of gentle waves coming in and out touching the pile.

And each wave in brings relaxation and each wave out carries a bit more of the sand away. Regardless how high the pile is, the power of the gentle waves is such that the pile becomes smaller and smaller—with each wave in bringing more relaxation and peace. With each wave out carrying more of the pile away, wave-by-wave, until the pile is gone. And *you* can just breathe in "strength" and "peace" with each inhalation, and with each exhalation *you* can truly say and think "calm." That's right.

When *you* are ready to formally leave this state of concentration *you* can do so by counting backwards from three to one. On three get ready, on two with *your* eyes closed roll up *your* eyes, and on one let *your* eyes open and take a deep breath and let it out. That will be the end of the formal exercise, but when *you* come out of it, *you* will still have the feeling of peace and comfort that *you* felt during it.

Ready, *three, two, one.*

Take a deep breath, and feel refreshed and proud about knowing how to help *yourself* at any time to feel calm, strong, and resourceful.

Option: Split Screen

Use all the sounds and noises to deepen *your* own experience and use only suggestions that are helpful for *you*. Resting *your* head and body comfortably *you* may proceed:

On *one*, do *one* thing: look up (pick any spot *you* like on the ceiling)

On *two*, do *two* things: slowly close *your* eyes and take a deep breath in.

On *three*, do *three* things: breathe out, relax the eyes, and let *your* body float.

... Good. Just imagine *your* whole body floating, floating with each breath easier and deeper right through where *you* are resting. Right now imagine that *you* are floating somewhere safe and comfortable, in a bath, a lake, a hot tub, or just floating in space, with each breath deeper and easier. With each breath in take in strength and with each breath out think "calm" and let go whatever there is to let go of. Just notice how with each breath *you* let a little more

143

tension out of your body as *you* let *your* whole body float, safe and comfortable; each breath deeper and easier.

... Just remaining in this state of concentration, focus on how *your* body is feeling right now. Where do *you* imagine *yourself* being? What is it like? Can *you* smell the air? Can *you* see what is around *you*? Good. Now this is *your* safe and pleasant place to be and *you* can use it in a sense to play a trick on whatever may happen and *you* can always return to it.

... *Your* concerns may have already drifted away and *you* may just enjoy the peace and delight at the place where *you* enjoy being. And if there are any worries left, and there may not be, *your* main job right now is to help *your* body feel comfortable. Remember, no matter what comes up, concentrate on *your* body floating. *You* can get uptight about things, but *your* body does not have to. Imagine that *you* are in this favorite spot. *You* may picture in *your* mind a screen like a movie screen or a TV screen or a piece of clear blue sky. First, *you* might see a pleasant scene on it. Now picture a large piece of blue screen divided in half. All right. Now on the left half, if there is still something that *you* are worrying about, picture that on the screen. Take *your* time to project it on the screen.

... When *you* are ready to proceed, move to the right side of the screen and picture what *you* will do about it. If *you* can't picture what *you* will do about it right now, just picture what *you* would recommend someone else do about it. *You* might be surprised at the solution *you* have to offer.

... Keep *your* body floating. If *you* are worrying about the outcome, it is okay, admit it to *yourself*, but *your* body does not have to get uptight about it. *You* may, but *your* body does not have to.

... Now *you* know that whatever happens there is always something *you* can do about it. And for now just concentrate on keeping *your* body floating and feeling safe and comfortable. That's right.

144

When *you* are ready to formally leave this state of concentration *you* can do so by counting backwards from three to one. On *three* get ready, on *two* with *your* eyes closed roll up *your* eyes, and on *one* let *your* eyes open and take a deep breath and let it out. That will be the end of the formal exercise, but when *you* come out of it, *you* will still have the feeling of peace and comfort that *you* felt during it.

Ready, *three, two, one*.

Take a deep breath, and feel refreshed and proud about knowing how to help *yourself* anytime to feel calm, strong, and resourceful.

Comfort Solution 8
Adjusting Body Functions and Symptoms to Your Advantage

Also see chapters 11, "Easing Pain," 13, "Affecting Blood Circulation and Body Functions," and 14, "Aiding Healing and Recovery."

CAUTION: *Managing medical symptoms should never be done without physician advice. For emergencies call 911 and/or use medication your physician prescribed.*

To further support yourself the following self-hypnosis techniques strategies can be used to help you influence your blood pressure, heart rate, breathing rate, and other vital body functions to improve your status. You can use them stand-alone or integrate them into the Basic Script presented in comfort solution 2, "Getting Started with Self-Hypnosis: the Basic Script." Sometimes just starting relaxation breathing can go a long way. (See comfort solution 1, "Relaxation Breathing Technique") Although for some of the following strategies, I give specific situations in which they were found to work well in clinical practice, the individual strategies are not limited to the examples given. You can mix and match, exchange, and use the same principles for whichever situation you want to influence.

Think of a situation to bring about the desired physiologic outcome

This strategy works quite well when one is too cold or too hot. The idea is to imagine a situation where your body naturally warms up agreeably and immerse yourself in the imagery. Perhaps a hot tub that you gradually enter to warm up just to the right degree, or anything that works well with the imagery you enjoy. On the other hand, if a hot flash overcomes you, focus on a pack of ice; imagine an arctic breeze, think of having your hands in a bucket of ice cold water and feel how it cools the circulating blood and makes you comfortable; make snow balls or whatever comes to mind. Always qualify that you want to warm up or cool down just to what is right for you. What this approach does is to either constrict the smallest vessels in your skin or open them widely to, respectively, keep body heat or dissipate it.

Learn about the mechanism of your symptom and suggest a solution

It helps to come up with a basic understanding of what you want to change. This strategy works well when something hurts or tightens up or gives you some other bothersome symptoms. In these settings, it helps to come up with an image that reflects the mechanism. You may ask your doctor about what is happening in the body causing the symptoms or read up about it. For example, say you know that when you travel in an airplane your ears tend to plug up on ascent and decent despite all precautions you have taken upfront. Instead of focusing on your hurt, focus on what causes the symptom and counteract its mechanism. Recall that air usually flows along a tiny canal between the inner ear and the mouth cavity and keeps the pressure in the ear in equilibrium; the canal is lined with delicate cells and when they swell just slightly with the change in cabin pressure air can't pass freely between the inner ear and mouth, which causes discomfort. If you think of these delicate cells that line the canal and focus hard to have them flatten and let air pass freely you may find yourself surprised how quickly the symptoms can resolve. This sequence can work in other situations, and the beauty is you don't even have to be absolutely correct about the mechanism—the main thing is that you attach an image to the process that functionally mirrors what is happening and find a solution.

Create an image of normal functioning

Sometimes it works well if you imagine how a system that works perfectly would look like and then communicate instructions to the system. The Hypnotherapy Group at the University Hospital of South Manchester, UK, uses such an approach successfully with patients with gut disorders and imparts the recommendation that "by allowing this image to be as strong and clear as possible, the more influence this will have over the gut." But you can easily replace gut with any other body system in question. The image can be close to the real thing or a metaphor that works for you. If the image of a cramp is that of a churning sea you can calm the waves, direct them to be coordinated and gentle and move the ships (a metaphor of your food) along just at the right speed, or whatever scenario works for you. Be creative. Let an image come up, and you may sometimes be amazed about the ingenuity of the mind. I personally once used the image of the electricity conducting bundle of my heart cells as a strand of fibers with increasingly strong insulation to prevent electric spoilers in their vicinity trying to enter and race up the heart beat when I had bouts of supraventricular tachycardia. As pointed above, this should not be your only means of diagnosis and treatment, but can be very helpful when one has to help oneself right here and now.

Create an image of healing

This strategy works well when dealing with immune responses and preparing for healing. Warts are considered an immune response to infection with the human papilloma virus and are well known to respond to hypnotic suggestions for healing. Medical treatment consists of icing, and because of this imagery of cooling the warts or of reducing their blood supply has been used successfully. However, others have been equally successful having the patients imagine an image of heat to shrink warts. The lesson here is that it is more important to come up with an image that is plausible to the individual rather than getting it physiologically correct. The image of healing can also be applied to closure of wounds with blood cells migrating into the area, sealing the gap, keeping it clean, secreting building materials that bridge the margins and strengthen the area, and making it blend in with the surrounding tissue. During recovery from chemotherapy thoughts of helping healthy blood cells being born, multiplying, and becoming strong could be another image of healing. These are just examples and you may have even better ideas of how the image should look.

Use dials

If you don't want to decide on imagery representing the system, you can imagine a control station in your brain with switches of your choice to adjust what you wish to adjust. It is important though that you are VERY specific and allow for the body's wisdom. Don't just say, "I want my heartbeat rate to go down;" instead engage the station controls to dial the heartbeat rate down safely, gently, and effortlessly to the desired number of beats per minute. Leave some room for your body's wisdom and definitely if you are not sure what the correct value would be suggest, "to a value that is best for me to function well." Focus on the dial while you are taking deep relaxing breaths. The method can also work well for managing pain by gradually dialing the pain sensation down from a current level to a manageable level.

Make long procedures seem shorter

Time distortion can happen naturally in a state of self-hypnosis with experienced time seemingly passing faster than on clock time. You can also make use of direct suggestions when you are concerned that a defined activity will inconvenience you for a longer stretch of time—for example having to keep your mouth open for a lengthy dental procedure or having to lie still for a a 3-hr imaging study. You can suggest yourself that "hours will pass like minutes, and minutes will pass like seconds."

Comfort Solution 9
Suggestions for Healing and Recovery

Also see chapter 14, "Aiding Healing and Recovery."

The following script, which can be used alone or integrated into the Basic Script (see comfort solution 2, "Getting Started with Self-Hypnosis: the Basic Script,") is designed to be most effective when read or listened to just prior to surgery, dentistry, or other treatment. The suggestions for aiding your recovery and healing that are featured in the script are called post-hypnotic suggestions because the effect of these suggestions extends beyond the end of the self-hypnotic session. The content of a *post-hypnotic suggestion* will depend largely on the goals you wish to achieve with the overall treatment. For example, you might insert suggestions to help you avoid undesirable side effects, and hasten your healing and recovery.

CAUTION: *While engaging in self-hypnotic relaxation do not drive or perform activities that requires your direct attention.*

NOTE: In the following Pre-Surgery Script, the introduction and reorientation parts (marked by a gray line running alongside the text) are modeled on the Basic Script in comfort solution 2, "Getting Started with Self-Hypnosis: the Basic Script." The unmarked text sections in between address several topics including easing discomfort and optimizing body functions. You can use just one, several, or all of the suggestions in the Pre-Surgery Script.

If you wish to design your own suggestions, refer to chapter 17, "Integrating Helpful Suggestions," for guidelines. The main thing to remember when constructing self-hypnosis script suggestions is to word them in positive terms that describe achievement of a normal body function. Do not word suggestions in negative terms that describe avoidance of a body malfunction. For example, it is better to suggest, "have a smooth transit of food through the intestines," rather than "not become constipated."

The introduction to the following Pre-Surgery Script is more extensive than the introduction that appears in the Basic Script because you may not want to reorient yourself before your procedure or surgery is completed or you may want to know how to enter a state of relaxation and leave it at any time. The script is easy to use and suitable for immediate use even if you didn't have time to read all the background in the book and just need support NOW.

CAUTION: *Before you begin, inquire as to what the conditions will be for you during the procedure so that your suggestions are appropriate. For example, ask if you will be allowed to drink, eat, or get up; and alter your suggestions to complement that reality.*

Pre-Surgery Script

Sometimes it helps to know how to help oneself to get through a medical procedure or any other experience more comfortably. It can be a way to help *your* body be more comfortable and also deal with any discomfort that might come up. It is just a form of concentration, like getting so caught up in a movie, a good book, or the Internet that *you* forget *you* are watching a movie, reading a book, or surfing the web. Just as with these experiences, *you* know that *you* are fully in control—*you* can close the book, switch the channel, or stop surfing whenever *you* want.

Now *you* may be curious about how *you* can use *your* imagination to enter a state of focused attention and physical relaxation. There are many ways to relax, but here is one simple way: Before starting *you* may want to know how to enter—and also to leave—

this state. This may come in handy when *you* want to watch what is happening during the procedure or when *you* will be recovering later in the hospital or at home. It is easy as 1-2-3: To relax

On *one*, do *one* thing, look up.

On *two*, *two* things, slowly close *your* eyes and take a deep breath.

On *three*, *three* things, breathe out, relax *your* eyes, and let *your* body float.

Okay, and when *you* are ready to return to the here and now, just count backwards from 3 to 1 while still bringing with *you* the feeling of comfort that *you* felt during it.

On *three*, *you* get ready,

on *two*, with *your* eyes closed *you* roll up *your* eyes,

and on *one*, *you* let *your* eyes open and take a deep breath in and let it out.

When ready to start, use all the sounds and noises to deepen *your* own experience and use only suggestions that are helpful for *you*. Resting *your* head and body comfortably, *you* may proceed:

On *one*, do *one* thing: look up (pick any spot *you* like on the ceiling)

On *two*, do *two* things: slowly close *your* eyes and take a deep breath in.

On *three*, do *three* things: breathe out, relax *your* eyes, and let *your* body float.

... Good. Just imagine *your* whole body floating, floating with each breath easier and deeper right through where *you* are resting. Right now imagine that *you* are floating somewhere safe and comfortable, in a bath, a lake, a hot tub, or just floating in space, with each breath deeper and easier. With each breath in, take in strength and with each breath out, think "calm" and let go of whatever there is to let go of. Just notice how with each breath *you* let a little more tension out of *your* body as *you* let *your* whole body float, safe and comfortable; each breath deeper and easier.

... Just remain in this state of concentration, focused on how *your* body is feeling right now. Where do *you* imagine *yourself* being? What is it like? Can *you* smell the air? Can *you* see what is around *you*? Good. Now this is *your* safe and pleasant place to be, and *you* can use it in a sense to play a trick on this whole surgery, treatment, or whatever is happening, and *you* can always return to it. *Your* body has to be here, but *you* don't.

... Now, if there is some discomfort, and there may be some, there is no point in fighting it. *You* can admit it, but then transform that sensation. If *you* feel some discomfort, *you* might find it helpful to make that part of *your* body feel warmer, as if *you* were in a bath. Or cooler—if that is more comfortable—as if *you* had ice or snow on that part of *your* body. This warmth and coolness becomes a protective filter between *you* and the pain. For now *you* can just enjoy remaining at the place of safety and enjoyment.

... It will be time to heal—and *your* body will know exactly what to do for *you* to become awake and fully aware of *your* surrounding; safely, gently, and effortlessly. *You* will know when the time is right to become fully awake again.

... And everything in *your* body will be working fine—just as it should be. *You* will be breathing on *your* own just as often and as deep as *you* want to and *you* need to.

... *You* will enjoy the air entering and leaving *your* lungs—just as often and deep as it needs to be. And *you* will enjoy how with each breath *you* get stronger.

... *You* can swallow the way *you* usually do and are probably going to want some water soon when it is appropriate. When the first sip of water wets *your* lips and mouth and throat it will find its way safely and gently into *your* stomach. And *you* will be able to swallow as *you* usually do and everything will be back to a good normal. *You* might even be hungry.

... When *you* are ready after *your* procedure, *you* will find it easy to empty *your* bladder. *You* might even be surprised at how quickly *your* body feels good. Just let the nurses know when *you* are ready.

... If needed, *you* can blow away any discomfort by taking some breaths and blowing them out. Or *you* can imagine putting an ice pack or warm pack on any spot that *you* want to feel more comfortable.

... And remember when people talk around *you*, and there are noises, listen only to what is helpful for *you*. Let the rest just go by and don't let it bother *you* at all. And *you* can set *your* body temperature just right.

... *You* will know when *your* procedure is completed and when the time is right for *you* to be ready and slowly, comfortably, and easily open *your* eyes and feel better than *you* did before. *You* will be very proud of *yourself* for having helped *yourself* so well through the procedure. It is good to know that *you* are a good boss for *your* body and can bring it safely and gently through all that happens. *You* know how to take care of *yourself* now and always.

> When *you* are ready to formally leave this state of concentration, *you* can do so by counting backwards from *three* to *one*. On *three*, get ready, on *two*, with *your* eyes closed roll up *your* eyes, and on *one*, let *your* eyes open and take a deep breath and let it out. That will be the end of the formal exercise, but when *you* come out of it, *you* will still have the feeling of peace and comfort that *you* felt during it.
>
> Ready, *three*, *two*, *one*.
>
> Take a deep breath, and feel refreshed and proud of knowing how to help *yourself* at any time to feel calm, strong, and resourceful.

Acknowledgments

I have had the great privilege, joy, and advantage to learn from many masters in the art of hypnotic language through personnel collaboration, participating in their training courses, obtaining their feedback, and reading their literature. I am particularly grateful to Drs. David Spiegel, Eleanor Laser, Barbara Barry, Max Shapiro, Steven Pauker, Dabney Ewin, and Donna Hamilton.

When it comes to actually making *Managing Your Medical Experience* happen, enormous credit and gratitude goes to Joan Lewis who keeps me on my toes, challenged and sane at the same time while giving her magic editorial touch. John Jenkins deserves sincere thanks for his expertise, patience and indulgence to bring my projects into just the right design. To Paul Senn, Graham Conway, Stasia Collins, Donna Wolfe, and Jim Stone I owe for their inspiration, enthusiasm, and continued support, and last, but the very most important, to Joe, my husband, for his love and support—making it all achievable and worthwhile.

References

Chapter 1

1. Lang EV, Berbaum KS, Lutgendorf SK. Large-core breast biopsy: Abnormal salivary cortisol profiles associated with uncertainty of diagnosis. Radiology 2009; 250:631-7.

2. Gustafsson O, Theorell T, Norming U, Perski A, Ohstrom M, Nyman CR. Psychological reactions in men screened for prostate cancer. British Journal of Urology 1995; 75:631-6.

3. Gustafsson O, Theorell T, Norming U, Perski A, Ohstrom M, Nyman CR. Psychological reactions in men screened for prostate cancer. British Journal of Urololgy 1995; 75:631-6.

4. Mishel MH. Uncertainty in illness. Image: The Journal of Nursing Scholarship 1988; 20:225-32.

5. Malone B. Direct patient access to lab results. Clinical Laboratory News [Internet]. 2012; 38. Available from: http://www.aacc.org/publications/cln/2012/april/Pages/PatientAccess.aspx

6. Beck M. New Rule grants patients direct access to lab results. Wall Street Journal. 2014; 4 February

Chapter 2

1. Lang, E. V., E. G. Benotsch, L. J. Fick, S. Lutgendorf, M. L. Berbaum, K. S. Berbaum, H. Logan, and D. Spiegel. 2000. Adjunctive non-pharmacologic analgesia for invasive medical procedures: A randomized trial. Lancet 355:1486-1490.

2. Lang, E. V., K. S. Berbaum, S. Faintuch, O. Hatsiopoulou, N. Halsey, X. Li, M. L. Berbaum, E. Laser, and J. Baum. 2006. Adjunctive self-hypnotic relaxation for outpatient medical procedures: A prospective randomized trial with women undergoing large core breast biopsy. Pain 126:155-164.

3. Lang, E. V., K. S. Berbaum, S. Paukur, S. Faintuch, G. M. Salazar, S. K. Lutgendorf, E. Laser, H. Logan, and D. Spiegel. 2008. Beneficial effects of hypnosis and adverse effects of empathic attention during percutaneous tumor treatment: When being nice does not suffice. Journal of Vascular and Interventional Radiology 19:897-905.

4. Flory, N., and E. V. Lang. 2011. Distress in the waiting room. Radiology 260:166-173.

5. Janis, I. L. 1958. Psychological stress: psychoanalytic and behavioral studies of surgical patients. New York: Wiley.

6. Briñol, P., and R. E. Petty. 2008. Embodied persuasion: Fundamental processes by which bodily responses can impact attitudes. In Embodiment

grounding: Social, cognitive, affective, and neuroscientific approaches, edited by G. R. Semin and E. R. Smith. Cambridge, England: Cambridge University Press.

7. Neumann, R., and F. Strack. 2000. "Mood contagion": The automatic transfer of mood between persons. Journal of Personality and Social Psychology 79:211-233.

8. Scott, D. W. 1983. Anxiety, critical thinking and information processing during and after breast biopsy. Nursing Research 32:24-28.

9. Beck, M. 2012. Anxiety can bring out the best. Wall Street Journal, 19 June, 2012, D1-D2.

10. Hay, J. L., K. D. McCaul, and R. E. Magnan. 2006. Does worry about breast cancer predict screening behavior? A meta-analysis of the prospective evidence. Preventive Medicine 42:401-408.

11. Spencer, S. M., and J. K. Norem. 1996. Reflection and distraction: Defensive pessimism, strategic optimism, and performance. Personality and Social Psychology Bulletin 22:354-365.

12. Andersen, B. L., and H. H. Tewfi. 1985. Psychological reactions to radiation therapy: Reconsiderations of the adaptive aspects of anxiety. Journal of Personality and Social Psychology 48:1024-1032.

13. Pham, L. B., and S. E. Taylor. 1999. From thought to action: Effects of process-versus outcome-based mental stimulations on performance. Personality and Social Psychology Bulletin 25:250-260.

14. Watkins, E. R. 2008. Constructive and unconstructive repetitive thought. Psychological Bulletin 134:163-206.

Chapter 3

1. Welch, H. G., L. M. Schwartz, and S. Woloshin. 2011. Overdiagnosed. Making people sick in the pursuit of health. Boston: Beacon Press.

2. Elwyn, G., D. O'Connell, D. Stacey, R. Volk, A. Edwards, A. Coulter, et al. 2006. Developing a quality criteria framework for patient decision aids: online international Delphi consensus process. British Medical Journal 333:417-423.

3. Stacey, D., C. I. Bennett, M. J. Barry, F. C. Nananda, K. B. Eden, M. Holmes-Rovner, et al. 2011. Decision aids for people facing health treatment and screening decisions. Edited by Cochrane Consumers and Communication Group, Intervention Review: John Wiley & Sons.

4. Elwyn, G., A. M. O'Connor, C. Bennett, R. G. Newcombe, M. Politi, A. M. Durand, et al. 2009. Assessing the quality of decision support technologies using the International Patient Decision Aid Standards instrument (IPDASi). PLOS One 4:1-9.

5. Consumer Reports. 2012. Privacy a casualty on Facebook. Boston Globe, 8 July, G2.

Chapter 4

1. Dijksterhuis, A. 2004. Think different: The merits of unconscious thought in preference development and decision making. Journal of Personality and Social Psychology 87:586-598.

2. Augusto, L. M. 2010. Unconscious knowledge: A survey. Advances in Cognitive Psychology 6:116-141.

3. Bechara, A., and A. R. Damasio. 2005. The somatic marker hypothesis: A neural theory of economic decision. Games and Economic Behavior 52:336-372.

4. Mikels, J. A., S. J. Maglio, A. E. Reed, and L. J. Kaplowitz. 2011. Should I go with my gut? Investigating the benefits of emotion-focused decision making. Emotion 11:743-753.

5. Bechara, A., H. Damasio, D. Tranel, and A. R. Damasio. 1996. Deciding advantageously before knowing the advantageous strategy. Science 275:1293-1295.

6. Cheek, D. B. 1994. Hypnosis: The application of ideomotor signals. Needham Heights, MA: Allyn and Bacon: A Division of Paramount Publishing.

7. Ewin, D. M., and B. N. Eimer. 2006. Ideomotor signals for rapid hypnoanalysis. Springfield, IL: Charles C. Thomas Publishers.

8. Lecron, L. M. 1964. Self-hypnotism; The technique and its use in daily living. Englewood Cliffs, NJ: Prentice-Hall, Inc.

9. Weitzenhofer, A. M. 1989. Ericksonian hypnotism: The Bandler/Grinder interpretation. In The practice of hypnotism. New York: John Wiley & Sons.

10. Rossi, E. L., and D. B. Cheek. 1988. Mind-body therapy. Methods of ideodynamic healing in hypnosis. New York: W. W. Norton.

Chapter 5

1. Skloot R. Henrietta's dance 2000 [April]. Available from: http://www.jhu.edu/~jhumag/0400web/01.html

2. Winslow R. Privacy deal over key set of genes. Wall Street Journal. 8 August 2013.

3. Ellis I, Mannion G, Warren-Jones A. Retained human tissues: a molecular genetics goldmine or modern grave robbing? A legal approach to obtaining and using stored human samples. Medical Law 2003; 22:357-72.

4. Hansson MG. Ethics and biobanks. British Journal of Cancer 2009; 100:8-12.

5. Helgesson G, Johnsson L. The right to withdraw consent to research on biobank samples. Medical Health Care Philosophy 2005; 8:315-21.

6. Girod J, Drabiak K. A proposal for comprehensive biobank research laws to promote translational medicine in Indiana. Indiana Health Law Review 2008; 5:217-50.

7. Turkow LP. Psychic consequences of loss and replacement of body parts. Journal of the American Psychoanalytical Association 1974; 22:170-81.

8. Goin MK, Goin JM, Gianini MH. The psychic consequences of a reduction mammaplasty. Plastic and Reconstructive Surgery 1977; 59:530-4.

9. Ewin DM, Eimer BN. Ideomotor signals for rapid hypnoanalysis. Springfield, IL: Charles C. Thomas Publishers; 2006.

10. Healthcare Environmental Resource Center. State-by-state regulated medical waste resource locator. Available from: http://www.hercenter.org/rmw/rmwlocator.cfm

11. Occupational Safety and Health Administration. Most Frequently Asked Questions Concerning the Bloodborne Pathogens Standard Occupational Safety and Health Act of 1970 (OSH Act) 19101030 1970.

Chapter 6

1. Neumann R, Strack F. "Mood contagion": The automatic transfer of mood between persons. Journal of Personality and Social Psychology 2000; 79:211-33.

2. Moss Kanter R. How winning streaks & losing streaks begin and end. New York: Crown Business; 2004.

Chapter 8

1. Garrett, P and J. Seidman ONC. "EMR vs EHR-What is the Difference?" http://www.healthit.gov/buzz-blog/electronic-health-and-medical-records/emr-vs-ehr-difference/.

2. HealthIT.gov. "Benefits of Health IT Information Technology in Health Care: The Next Consumer Revolution," http://www.healthit.gov/patients-families/benefits-health-it.

3. HealthIT.gov. "How can I access my health information/medial record?" http://www.healthit.gov/patients-families/benefits-health-it.

Chapter 9

1. Berglund B, Lindvall T, Schwela DH. Guidelines for community noise1999 21 March 2014. Available from: http://www.who.int/docstore/peh/noise/guidelines2.html.

2. Busch-Vishniac IJ, West JE, Barnhill C, Hunter T, Orellana D, Chivukula R. Noise levels in Johns Hopkins Hospital. The Journal of the Acoustical Society of America 2005; 118:3629-45.

3. Cmiel CA, Karr DM, Gasser DM, Oliphant LM, Neveau AJ. Noise control: a nursing team's approach to sleep promotion. The American journal of nursing 2004; 104:40-8; quiz 8-9.

4. Kracht JM, Busch-Vishniac IJ, West JE. Noise in the operating rooms of Johns Hopkins Hospital. The Journal of the Acoustical Society of America 2007; 121:2673-80.

5. McLaren E, Maxwell-Armstrong C. Noise pollution on an acute surgical ward. Annals of the Royal College of Surgeons of England 2008; 90:136-9.

6. National Institute on Deafness and Other Communication Disorders (NI-DCD). Common sounds 2010 [updated 7 June 2010 21 March 2014]. Available from: https://http://www.nidcd.nih.gov/health/education/teachers/pages/common_sounds.aspx.

7. Konkani A, Oakley B, Bauld TJ. Reducing hospital noise: a review of medical device alarm management. Biomedical instrumentation & technology / Association for the Advancement of Medical Instrumentation 2012; 46:478-87.

8. Perez-Cruz P, Nguyen L, Rhondali W, Hui D, Palmer JL, Sevy I, et al. Attitudes and perceptions of patients, caregivers, and health care providers toward background music in patient care areas: an exploratory study. Journal of palliative medicine 2012; 15:1130-6.

9. Cooke M, Chaboyer W, Hiratos MA. Music and its effect on anxiety in short waiting periods: a critical appraisal. Journal of Clinical Nursing 2005; 14:145-55.

10. Kain ZN, Caldwell-Andrews AA, Krivutza DM, Weinberg ME, Gaal D, Wang SM, et al. Interactive music therapy as a treatment for preoperative anxiety in children: a randomized controlled trial. Anesth Analg 2004; 98:1260-6, table of contents.

11. Stevenson RA, Schlesinger JJ, Wallace MT. Effects of divided attention and operating room noise on perception of pulse oximeter pitch changes: a laboratory study. Anesthesiology 2013; 118:376-81.

Chapter 10

1. Hauser W, Hansen E, Enck P. Nocebo phenomena in medicine: their relevance in everyday clinical practice. Deutsches Arzteblatt international 2012; 109:459-65.

2. Colloca L, Miller FG. The nocebo effect and its relevance for clinical practice. Psychosomatic Medicine 2011; 73:598-603.

3. Spiegel H. Nocebo: The power of suggestibility. Preventive Medicine 1997; 26:616-21.

4. Cocco G. Erectile dysfunction after therapy with metoprolol: the Hawthorne effect. Cardiology 2009; 112:174-7.

5. Lang EV, Hatsiopoulou O, Koch T, Lutgendorf S, Kettenmann E, Logan H, et al. Can words hurt? Patient-provider interactions during invasive medical procedures. Pain 2005; 114:303-9.

6. Varelmann D, Pancaro C, Cappiello EC, Camann WR. Nocebo-induced hyperalgesia during local anesthetic injection. Anesthesia & Analgesia 2010; 110:868-70.

Chapter 11

1. Bayer TL, Coverdale JH, Chiang E, Bangs M. The role of prior pain experience and expectancy in psychologically and physically induced pain. Pain 1998; 74:327-31.

2. Lang EV, Benotsch EG, Fick LJ, Lutgendorf S, Berbaum ML, Berbaum KS, et al. Adjunctive non-pharmacologic analgesia for invasive medical procedures: A randomized trial. Lancet 2000; 355:1486-90.

3. Lang EV, Tan G, Amihai I, Jensen MP. Analyzing acute procedural pain in clinical trials. Pain 2014:in press.

4. Lang EV, Berbaum KS, Pauker S, Faintuch S, Salazar GM, Lutgendorf SK, et al. Beneficial effects of hypnosis and adverse effects of empathic attention during percutaneous tumor treatment: When being nice does not suffice. Journal of Vascular and Interventional Radiology 2008; 19:897-905.

5. Lee JS, Pyun YD. Use of hypnosis in the treatment of pain. The Korean Journal of Pain 2012; 25:75-80.

6. Lang EV, Berbaum KS, Faintuch S, Hatsiopoulou O, Halsey N, Li X, et al. Adjunctive self-hypnotic relaxation for outpatient medical procedures: A prospective randomized trial with women undergoing large core breast biopsy. Pain 2006; 126:155-64 PMCID: PMC2656356.

7. Lang EV, Berbaum KS, Lutgendorf SK. Large-core breast biopsy: Abnormal salivary cortisol profiles associated with uncertainty of diagnosis. Radiology 2009; 250:631-7.

8. Faymonville ME, Fissette J, Mambourg PH, Roediger L, Joris J, Lamy M. Hypnosis as adjunct therapy in conscious sedation for plastic surgery. Regional Anesthesia 1995; 20:145-51.

9. Montgomery GH, Bovbjerg DH, Schnur JB, David D, Goldfarb A, Weltz CR, et al. A randomized clinical trial of a brief hypnosis intervention to control side effects in breast surgery patients. Journal of the National Cancer Institute 2007; 99:1304-12.

10. Patterson DR, Questad KA, de Lateur BJ. Hypnotherapy as an adjunct to narcotic analgesia for the treatment of pain for burn debridement. The American Journal of Clinical Hypnosis 1989; 31:156-63.

11. Flory N, Salazar GM, Lang EV. Hypnosis for acute distress management during medical procedures. The International Journal of Clinical and Experimental Hypnosis 2007; 55:303-17.

12. Montgomery GH, David D, Winkel G, Silverstein JH, Bovberg DH. The effectiveness of adjunctive hypnosis with surgical patients: A meta-analysis. Anesthesia and Analgesia 2002; 94:1639-45.

13. Lang EV, Yuh WT, Ajam A, Kelly R, Macadam L, Potts R, et al. Understanding patient satisfaction ratings for radiology services. AJR American Journal of Roentgenology 2013; 201:1190-5; quiz 6.

14. Faintuch S, Collares FB, Salazar GMM, Lang EV. Nontraditional pain mangement in interventional radiology. In: Ray CE, editor. Pain management in interventional radiology. Cambridge: Cambridge University Press; p. 280-95.

162

Chapter 12

1. Flory N, Lang E. Distress in the radiology waiting room. Radiology 2011; in press.

2. Lang EV, Benotsch EG, Fick LJ, Lutgendorf S, Berbaum ML, Berbaum KS, et al. Adjunctive non-pharmacologic analgesia for invasive medical procedures: A randomized trial. Lancet 2000; 355:1486-90.

3. Lang EV, Berbaum KS, Faintuch S, Hatsiopoulou O, Halsey N, Li X, et al. Adjunctive self-hypnotic relaxation for outpatient medical procedures: A prospective randomized trial with women undergoing large core breast biopsy. Pain 2006; 126:155-64 PMCID: PMC2656356.

4. Lang EV, Berbaum KS, Pauker S, Faintuch S, Salazar GM, Lutgendorf SK, et al. Beneficial effects of hypnosis and adverse effects of empathic attention during percutaneous tumor treatment: When being nice does not suffice. Journal of Vascular and Interventional Radiology 2008; 19:897-905.

5. Schupp C, Berbaum KS, Berbaum ML, Lang EV. Pain and anxiety during interventional radiological procedures. Effect of patients' state anxiety at baseline and modulation by nonpharmacologic analgesia adjuncts Journal of Vascular and Interventional Radiology 2005; 16:1585-92.

6. Lang EV, Chen F, Fick LJ, Berbaum KS. Determinants of intravenous conscious sedation for arteriography. Journal of Vascular and Interventional Radiology 1998; 9:407-12.

7. Wood Brooks A. Get excited: Reappraising pre-perfomance anxiety as excitement. Journal of Experimental Psychology [Internet]. 2013: [1-15 pp.]. Available from: http://www.apa.org/pubs/journals/releases/xge-a0035325.pdf.

8. Kabat-Zinn J. Full catastrophe living. Using the wisdom of your body and mind to face stress, pain, and illness. New York: Delta Book; 1990 p. 132-9.

9. Gerschman JA. Dental anxiety disorders, phobias and hypnotizability. In: Burrow DG, Stanley RO, Bloom PB, editors. International Handbook of Clinical Hypnosis: John Wiley & Sons Ltd; 2001 p. 299-307.

Chapter 13

1. Lang EV, Benotsch EG, Fick LJ, Lutgendorf S, Berbaum ML, Berbaum KS, et al. Adjunctive non-pharmacologic analgesia for invasive medical procedures: A randomized trial. Lancet 2000;355: 1486-90.

2. Lang EV, Berbaum KS, Pauker S, Faintuch S, Salazar GM, Lutgendorf SK, et al. Beneficial effects of hypnosis and adverse effects of empathic attention during percutaneous tumor treatment: When being nice does not suffice. Journal of Vascular and Interventional Radiology 2008; 19:897-905.

3. Lang EV, Berbaum KS, Faintuch S, Hatsiopoulou O, Halsey N, Li X, et al. Adjunctive self-hypnotic relaxation for outpatient medical procedures: A prospective randomized trial with women undergoing large core breast biopsy. Pain 2006; 126:155-64

4. DeBenedittis G, Cigada M, Bianchi A, Signorini MG, Cerutti S. Autonomic changes during hypnosis: A heart rate variability power spectrum analysis as a marker of sympathico-vagal balance. International Journal of Clinical and Experimental Hypnosis 1994; 42:140-52.

5. Hippel CV, Hole G, Kaschka WP. Autonomic profile under hypnosis as assessed by heart rate variability and spectral analysis. Pharmacopsychiatry 2001; 34:111-3.

6. Anderson JL, Horne BD. Nonlinear heart rate variability. Journal of Cardiovascular Electrophysiology 2005; 16:21-3.

7. Stein P, Domitrovich PP, Huikuri HV, Kleiger RE, for the CAST Investigators. Traditional and nonlinear heart rate variability are each independently associated with mortality after myocardial infarction. Journal of Cardiovascular Electrophysiology 2005; 16:13-20.

Chapter 14

1. Ginandes C, Brooks P, Sando W, Jones C, Aker J. Can medical hypnosis accelerate post-surgical wound healing? Results of a clinical trial. The American Journal of ClinicalHhypnosis 2003; 45:333-51.

2. Ginandes CS, Rosenthal DI. Using hypnosis to accelerate the healing of bone fractures: a randomized controlled pilot study. Alternative Therapies in Health and Medicine 1999; 5:67-75.

Chapter 15

1. Fick LJ, Lang EV, Logan HL, Lutgendorf S, Benotsch EG. Imagery content during nonpharmacologic analgesia in the procedure suite: Where your patients would rather be. Academic Radiology 1999; 6:457-63.

2. Blankfield RP. Suggestion, relaxation, and hypnosis as adjuncts in the care of surgery patients: A review of the literature. American Journal of Clinical Hypnosis 1991; 33:172-86.

3. Ewin DM, Eimer BN. Ideomotor signals for rapid hypnoanalysis. Springfield, IL: Charles C. Thomas Publishers; 2006.

4. Hoeft F, Gabrieli JDE, Whitfield-Gabrieli S, Haas BW, Bammer R, Vinod M, et al. Functional Brain Basis of Hypnotizability. Arch Gen Psychiatry 2012; 69:1064-72.

5. Spiegel H, Spiegel D. Trance and treatment: Clinical uses of hypnosis. New York: Basic Books; 1978.

6. Montgomery GH, David D, Winkel G, Silverstein JH, Bovberg DH. The effectiveness of adjunctive hypnosis with surgical patients: A meta-analysis. Anesthesia and Analgesia 2002; 94:1639-45.

7. DiClementi JD, Deffenbaugh J, Jackson D. Hypnotizability, absorption and negative cognitions as predictors of dental anxiety: two pilot studies. Journal of the American Dental Association 2007; 138:1242-50.

Chapter 16

1. Braid J. Neurypnology, or the rationale of nervous sleep, considered with animal magnetism. London: J. Churchill; 1843.

2. Bramwell JM. Hypnotism. Its history, practice and theory. . London: Alexander Moring Ltd; 1906. 283 p.

3. Olness K, Kohen DP. Hypnosis and hypnotherapy with children. Third edition. New York London: The Guilford Press; 1996.

4. Wells WR. Experiments in waking hypnosis for instructional purposes. Journal of Abnormal and Social Psychology 1924;18:389-404.

5. Wark D. Alert hypnosis. A review and case report. American Journal of Clincal Hypnosis 2006;48:291-300.

6. Wark D, laPlante PM. Reading in alert state: Effect on comprehension. Hypnos 1991;17:90-7.

7. Capofons A, Mendoza ME. "Waking" hypnosis in clincial practice. In: Lynn SJ, Rhue JW, Kirsch i, editors. Handbook of clinical hypnosis. 2nd edition. Washington, DC: American Psychological Association; 2010. p. 293-317.

Chapter 17

1. Wark, D. 2006. Alert hypnosis. A review and case report. American Journal of Clincal Hypnosis. 48:291-300.

2. Wark, D., and P. M. laPlante. 1991. Reading in alert state: Effect on comprehension. Hypnos. 17:90-97.

3. Hammond, C. C. 1992. Manual for self-hypnosis: The American Society of Clinical Hypnosis.

About the Author

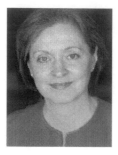

Elvira V. Lang, MD, PhD, FSIR, FSCEH, is an award-winning interventional radiologist acclaimed for her pioneer research on the clinical effectiveness and efficiency of pre- and intra- procedural hypnotic interventions. Dr. Lang is featured extensively in the popular press and on television, and is recognized internationally as leading expert in the use of self-hypnotic relaxation during medical procedures. Her research-based refinement of the way medical personnel interacts with patients has resulted in greater patient comfort, better outcomes, and shortened duration of medical procedures.

Dr. Lang has held faculty positions at the University of Heidelberg, Stanford University, the University of Iowa, and Harvard Medical School. An avid advocate of the need for scientific proof to back proposed healthcare procedure changes, she is a prolific researcher; her research work has been acknowledged with the Ernest R. Hilgard Award for Scientific Excellence for a Lifetime of Published Experimental Work.

Her research team was awarded substantive government funding to test the effects of nonpharmacologic management of pain and distress in clinical settings. Dr. Lang's team demonstrated in three large-scale prospective randomized studies with more than 700 patients that self-hypnotic relaxation on the procedure table reduces pain, anxiety, drug use, and complications. This research experience began a process that culminated in the refined formulation of Comfort Talk®, her proprietary non-pharmaceutical process that empowers patients to experience their medical encounters with greater comfort and control.

Through her publications and efforts as Past President of the New England Society of Clinical Hypnosis and the Society of Clinical and Experimental Hypnosis, Dr. Lang promoted the training in Comfort Talk® for nurses and licensed healthcare professionals within the scope of their practice including MRI, breast care, oncology, urology, gastroenterology, diagnostic and interventional radiology, obstetrics, and dentistry. To facilitate this training Dr. Lang co-authored the book *Patient Sedation Without Medication*—a how-to guide for medical personnel. The response to this publication and feedback from patients led her to write *Managing Your Medical Experience,* which puts the knowledge of how to navigate the modern healthcare system as well as the healing, calming power of self-hypnosis directly in patients' hands.

Explore Comfort Talk®

Check the Foundation

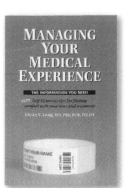

The strategies and step-by-step self-hypnosis techniques presented in *Managing Your Medical Experience* for patients, grew from author Elvira Lang, MD's extensive research and field testing of Comfort Talk® Training—a training system that provides medical professionals with the knowledge and skills needed to help patients tap into their mind's natural ability to block pain and reduce stress. *For more information about Comfort Talk®, our training sites, and news please visit* **www.hypnalgesics.com**

Sample the Professional Perspective

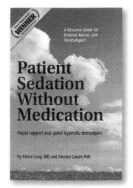

Managing Your Medical Experience—designed for personal use by patients—contains refined versions of the same techniques presented in Dr. Lang's co-authored book for medical professionals. *To sample the professional version of Comfort Talk®, purchase* Patient Sedation Without Medication *at* **www.hypnalgesics.com/pages/pr.Book.html**

Tune In

The Comfort Solution scripts in *Managing Your Medical Experience* are constructed on the assumption that someone will read the script aloud to the self-hypnosis subject or that the subject will make a recording of the script to play when desired. Also available is an

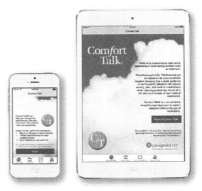

app with customizable audio recordings. *Download the Comfort Talk® app from the Apple Store or through:* **www.hypnalgesics.com/pages/p.Resources.App.html**

Stay Up-to-Date

Dr. Lang and the Hypnalgesic team work at the cutting edge of research, development, and education in patient comfort. *To keep informed of the discoveries, events, and opportunities that continue to emerge, sign-up for our quarterly newsletter at* **www.hypnalgesics.com/pages/ p.Resources.Newsletter.html**

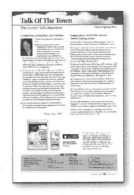

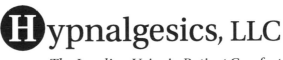

ⓗypnalgesics, LLC
The Leading Voice in Patient Comfort

Made in the USA
Charleston, SC
30 July 2014